FOOD STORAGE
FOR PREPPERS

A Week-By-Week Plan for
Surviving an Apocalypse

David Nash

Skyhorse Publishing

Skyhorse Publishing books may be purchased in bulk at special discounts for sales promotion, corporate gifts, fund-raising, or educational purposes. Special editions can also be created to specifications. For details, contact the Special Sales Department, Skyhorse Publishing, 307 West 36th Street, 11th Floor, New York, NY 10018 or info@skyhorsepublishing.com.

Skyhorse® and Skyhorse Publishing® are registered trademarks of Skyhorse Publishing, Inc.®, a Delaware corporation.

Visit our website at www.skyhorsepublishing.com.

10 9 8 7 6 5 4 3 2 1

Library of Congress Cataloging-in-Publication Data is available on file.

Cover design by Kai Texel

Print ISBN: 978-1-5107-6826-0
Ebook ISBN: 978-1-5107-7007-2

Printed in China

Table of Contents

Projects

Dedication

This book is dedicated to my son William Tell Nash. As he grows into manhood, I wish him to learn the lesson that food storage and other self-reliance actions are not done out of fear.

We prepare with self-discipline because we value personal responsibility, and because we prefer to be producers rather than moochers.

I hope he never has to live solely on our food storage, but I intend for him to be able to.

Foreword

He promotes persistence as opposed to one great event.

He promotes consistency in self-sufficiency rather than some survivalist, hermit philosophy.

Prepare for what's to come—his persistence continues in this work, so important that it taunted the author for a place in his broad array of published works until he finally relented and gave this topic the dedicated platform it deserved.

The book is important and significant because . . .

If I ever needed a macho superhero type of character in my camp, it would be David Nash—but don't let that hardcore exterior fool you. This book officially removes his manly mask and exposes him as a mushy ole teddy bear underneath.

Everybody knows that good food is the way to win someone's heart as it's one of the best expressions of love. So while you may have seen his Rambo-like persona in David's previously published works involving firearms, street smart self-defense, or chasing and hunting down your next batch of homemade sausage, make no mistake about it: David has set out to woo you with his passion for delicious meals regardless of the circumstances in which you may find yourself. Alien invasion, a massive earthquake, or the next world war? No problem! David is determined and persistent in promoting his passion for all the ways you can enjoy a great meal.

While it's critical for survival, health, and emotional well-being, food is also about love. In this work, David guides you through fifty-two clever ways that you can create delicious, nurturing, comforting, and realistic dishes in the midst of any kind of a scenario. While freeze-dried food manufacturers would have you believe that spending your kid's college fund is necessary in order to avoid starvation someday soon, David lives confidently at the other end of the spectrum, spreading lots of passion amidst his plethora of ideas and projects that can help anyone to look forward to mealtime—even if it means camping amidst the ruins of your own home.

For those who consider themselves "preppers," David has a special message for you. Often, he has seen so many who deliberately "prepare" for nothing but misery as they half-heartedly "plan" on eating lackluster, energy-sucking, immune-crashing substances that can barely be considered "food." David is wise in his understanding that a crisis is obviously rough enough without you deliberately planning to suffer through an unpleasant meal or two on top of it. So, through these fifty-two projects he teaches you how you can easily take affordable steps *now* to ensure that your mealtime will be the least of your worries tomorrow. In fact, he shows how simple planning and efforts now will serve you well physically, emotionally, and, perhaps, even financially later on down the road.

In the book's introduction, David encourages folks to *use* the book to the point of getting flour and juice on the pages. But I discovered that if you truly utilize this valuable resource properly, you'll no doubt end up with signs of wear and tear thanks to great delights such as velvety caramel, creamy butter, heavenly bacon, and mouthwatering corn cob jelly, which David cleverly creates using parts that most people would throw down the drain or into the trash.

Make no mistake about it, David is a real person. He's busier than a one-armed paperhanger just like the rest of us and doesn't have time or tolerance for lengthy processes that feel like they require a doctorate in physics. His no-nonsense approach to these projects is sure to endear the busiest of moms, while still being man enough to earn Dad a gold star or two. David takes his reality one step further by ensuring that his projects are doable regardless of the size of your bank account; he clearly prefers the "do-it-yourself" methods over those "spending-gobs-of-money-on-items-that-will-only-collect-dust-in-the-basement-until-there's-an-apocalypse—at-which-time-you're-likely-to-forget-you-even-had-such-items" type of methods. (*Yes,* he says, you *can* make delicious homemade pasta without the fancy equipment!)

In the interest of making every opportunity for a good meal realistic for everyone, David walks you through multiple methods to accomplish your goals so you have plenty of options to choose from! That's my kind of "prepper"—one who uses multipurpose tools *and* methods to go along with the multipurpose tangible items!

Whether it's discussing nuances of browning a dish more beautifully with honey, or confessing to ruining his wife's treasured appliances a time or two, you'll find yourself fully engaged in what he has to teach you. I suspect that rather than feeling overwhelmed with another list of "everything that needs to be done for mealtime sanity amidst a crisis," you'll find David's enthusiasm contagious and find yourself feeling like his projects are a moment of peaceful respite for you!

Unfortunately, there is a downside to partaking of David's passion-driven projects; they really get in the way of that afternoon you had planned to watch the *Gilligan's Island* marathon in order to glean Self-Sufficiency 101 Training. So be warned that once David entices you to venture into the "doing" of these

Introduction to the 2021 Edition

2020 was quite an eventful year for most of us. As I sit and write an introduction to my re-released prepper food book, I am listening to the news describe massive power outages and ice storms in Texas, large scale under or un-employment, fear of communicable diseases, and general societal discontent.

It is this kind of unrest and uncertainty that lead me to general personal preparedness. While some look at the term prepper as a pejorative term describing what some may want to see as a socially inept paranoid loner, I see preppers with a different view. In my experience, a prepper is someone with the common sense to know the world doesn't play fair. With that knowledge a prepper has the wisdom and discipline to sacrifice in the short term to thrive during harder times.

Having food security brings peace of mind. I don't believe in zombies, but I do see the price of food rising faster than the many paychecks. Government quarantine may prevent your normal grocery run. Social unrest may make travel unsafe. Or like the current ice storm situation, weather may cause electricity outages or make travel impossible.

Luckily for my family, in 2020 we were able to finally buy a family farm, and one of the first things we did was raise a couple of feeder hogs and a LOT of meat chickens. So, as I watch the unrest, my family benefits from the safety net of a couple of freezers full of meat. I understand that not everyone can (or wants to) raise their own food. Raising your own animals for slaughter is not easy and it sure isn't cheaper than large-scale factory farming. However, even if you don't produce your own food, you can still gain a large measure of food security with a well-thought-out food storage plan.

I authored this book while my family lived in a suburban neighborhood. Our situation at the time limited what we could produce in the garden and backyard menagerie. Within the chapters inside, you can find workable techniques to preserve and store (and even cook) foodstuffs, no matter if you buy it, grow it, or raise it. Everything in this book works, and I gained a couple inches around the midsection proving it in my own kitchen. My hope for you is that you and those your care about never go hungry and that this book helps in that in some small way.

David Nash
DGW Homestead

Introduction

I really don't like the term "prepper." Recently, it seems to have acquired a slightly pejorative connotation—basically "survivalist–lite." In response to this, I have stolen terminology from my past work in governmental emergency management and call what I do "advocating for a disaster-resilient lifestyle."

In reality it doesn't matter what we modern folks call it. Prepping is nothing new—historically it has just been called "good common sense." For thousands of years, humans have known that seasons change, crops fail, volcanoes sometimes explode, and that the tribes that thrive learn the most efficient means to store food.

In statistics, there is a term called regression to the mean (or reversion to mediocrity) in which short-term measurements can fluctuate widely (test scores, stocks, climate); however, when looked at over time the measurements actually stabilize. What that means to us disaster-minded folks is that no matter how great we are doing today or how bad it seems, neither good nor bad times will last. The common sense thing to do in this scenario is to put resources aside when we have plenty to create a cushion for times when we don't have enough.

When I meet with other preparedness advocates, I am always amazed at the vast differences in how each individual solves common problems. I have met those who plan to "bug out" and live the life of a mountain man, engineers who have triple redundant technological systems in place to reduce dependence on grid-supplied utilities, off-grid families that reduce their lives to simplicity and try to produce the majority of their own staples, and other confused guys like me who cannot seem to find a preference, but who rather borrow bits and pieces from everyone we meet.

In the end the commonality is that we all need food, water, and shelter—everything else is just a nicety to have.

When writing my earlier book *52 Prepper Projects* (Skyhorse Publishing, 2013), I had to cut out several food-related projects to provide a balanced collection. In this book, I am getting back to basics and focusing entirely on food. This book has an emphasis on food preservation rather than production because, while not everyone has the resources needed to produce the majority of their own food, everyone reading this does have access to the neighborhood grocery store.

How to Use This Book

Like *52 Prepper Projects*, this book is loosely based on the premise that the reader will pick one project a week, and that the projects in the beginning of the book are simpler and provide the foundation for the more complex projects in the later pages.

However, as I research projects, I find that reading about something is different than actually doing it. So, earlier projects may seem harder than later projects. I also find that everyone has a different point of view and skill level.

While the book is intended to be organized in a manner to make it easier on the reader to work on projects consecutively, I think most people will jump around and complete projects as they need or want to do them. At my house, we do projects based on the blessings of both the good idea fairy, or if I see something in the grocery store that reminds me of a certain project . . .

No matter how you complete the projects in the book, this is not designed to be a cool book sitting on the shelf. Reading is a poor substitute for doing.

Get flour on the cover and juice stains on the inner pages—dog-eared and used or creased books are usually owned by smarter people.

Lastly, I want you to understand that I have researched, studied, and completed each of these projects—multiple times each. But your results may vary, so adjust accordingly based on your own judgment, needs, and skills. In the end, this book is designed to help you help yourself. In the words of the famous naturalist James Audubon, "When the bird and the book disagree, always believe the bird."

Food Safety Issues

Food safety can be a contentious issue. Some demand perfectly safe techniques, while others eschew modern safety and stick with their secret family recipe because "Granny did it this way her whole life and never got sick."

Personally, I prefer to use common sense. The various extension office standards and those that come from the National Center for Home Food Preservation are deemed safe because, if you follow their techniques perfectly, no food-borne pathogens can survive their canning process.

Due to their strict methods, things like butter (canned ghee), eggs, or cheeses cannot be "safely" canned. This is because botulism spores may be able to survive in the center of the can. However, any homesteader or prepper who follows Internet blogs is bound to have found several websites that show people canning butter, eggs, or cheese.

I have canned and seen others can items that the powers that be have deemed unsafe. That doesn't mean you should do so. You can die from improperly canned foods.

For the record, I would caution anyone who wants to can to strictly follow the extension office standards and official recipes. This is the only way to ensure that you do not die of slow paralysis brought on by the botulism toxin.

I would also like to educate the reader on botulism poisoning—especially since 48 of the 116 cases of botulism poisoning in the United States from 1996 to 2008 were caused by improperly home canned vegetables.

First off, botulism is a bacterium called *Clostridium botulinum* that lives in the soil. When either the bacteria itself or the harder-to-kill spores are sealed in the proper environment, they grow and produce a toxin that even in tiny amounts can cause paralysis and death.

Of course for botulism to occur you need:

- Anaerobic conditions (no oxygen)
- Temperatures above 39°F
- Moisture
- pH greater than 4.6
- In almost any home canned item you will create the first three conditions.

In case you aren't familiar, the terms "acid" and "base" are ways to describe the properties of a chemical, similar to water that is "hot" or "cold." While mixing hot and cold water forms warm water, mixing acids and bases will even out the pH level. A substance that is neither acidic nor basic is called "neutral."

The pH scale measures the range of how acidic or basic a material is. It ranges from 0 to 14. A pH of 7 is neutral. Water is a 7 on the pH chart.

A pH less than 7 is acidic, and a pH greater than 7 is basic. Each point on the pH chart grows by ten times. So, a pH of 3 is ten times more acidic than something with a pH of 4 and 100 times (10 x 10) more acidic than something with a pH of 5. The same holds true for bases.

A low pH kills botulism spores, which is the reason why we don't have to pressure can food with a high level of acidity. On the other hand, I know many people who think you don't have to pressure can pickled items, since vinegar is an acid. However, in many cases (especially pickled eggs), the pH level at the center of the food item can remain unchanged. So, *if* botulism is present, bacteria would grow in the center and create the toxin in the yolk of a pickled egg, even if the rest of the egg is of the proper pH to kill botulism.

I would like to caution you to be careful. If you doubt the safety of any preserved foods, throw it out. This is especially important if the food has the following signs, which indicate contamination:

• Bulging, leaking, or swollen cans
• Damaged or cracked containers
• If the can spurts liquid or foam when opened
• If the food is moldy, off colored, or smells bad

All this may seem difficult or confusing, but it is a vital part of learning how to properly can food. I was a little "fast and loose" with canning until I ate some home canned food and got it in my head that I should have been more cautious (after I had eaten it). I spent a long weekend checking myself for the initial symptoms of botulism poisoning and have since been very careful to pay close attention to detail.

$10 Weekly Food Storage Program

Food storage does not have to be difficult or break the bank. I cannot afford to buy prepackaged yearly supplies of freeze-dried premium foods. However, not being able to spend tens of thousands of dollars in food does not keep me from providing for my family.

Instead of sprinting toward a nonexistent finish line of "preparedness," I prefer to move in a reasoned and steady pace, building up my stores slowly and without causing marital discord.

While I live by what I write, some projects I write about are things I tried a couple times out of curiosity or because I wanted to gain a basic skill. This particular program is a staple of my emergency plan, and is how I have gotten to the level of preparedness that I am in currently.

What my family does is to make a shopping list of what we need for the week, and buy a little extra each week. $10 (or $5 or $25 depending on your budget) may not seem much, but over time it comes up to a substantial amount of food. An extra $10 constitutes ten more cans of vegetables or several pounds of dried beans.

We found that after obtaining and storing several months' worth of the foods we eat daily, we were able to skip our normal grocery trip and buy larger amounts of food in bulk for the same price. Over time we even saved enough to make bulk purchases of meats.

If you want some help deciding what to purchase, the list below is a good representation of one full year of food for two adults.

It would be a simple process to begin with week one and get that week's food item while you are doing your normal shopping.

1. 6 Pounds of Salt
2. 5 Cans Cream of Chicken Soup
3. 20 Pounds of Sugar
4. 8 Cans Tomato Soup
5. 50 Pounds of Wheat
6. 6 Pounds of Macaroni
7. 20 Pounds of Sugar
8. 8 Cans of Tuna

9. 6 Pounds of Yeast
10. 50 Pounds of Wheat
11. 8 Cans of Tomato Soup
12. 20 Pounds of Sugar
13. 10 Pounds of Powdered Milk
14. 7 Boxes of Macaroni and Cheese
15. 50 Pounds of Wheat
16. 5 Cans of Cream of Chicken Soup
17. 1 Bottle of 500 Multi-Vitamins
18. 10 Pounds of Powdered Milk
19. 5 Cans of Cream of Mushroom Soup
20. 50 Pounds of Wheat
21. 8 Cans of Tomato Soup
22. Pounds of Sugar
23. 8 Cans of Tuna
24. 6 Pounds of Shortening
25. 50 Pounds of Wheat
26. 5 Pounds of Honey
27. 10 Pounds of Powdered Milk
28. 20 Pounds of Sugar
29. 5 Pounds of Peanut Butter
30. 50 Pounds of Wheat
31. 7 Boxes of Macaroni and Cheese
32. 10 Pounds of Powdered Milk
33. 1 Bottle of 500 Aspirin
34. 5 Cans of Cream of Chicken Soup
35. 50 Pounds of Wheat
36. 7 Boxes of Macaroni and Cheese
37. 6 Pounds of Salt
38. 20 Pounds of Sugar
39. 8 Cans of Tomato Soup
40. 50 Pounds of Wheat
41. 5 Cans of Cream of Chicken Soup
42. 20 Pounds of Sugar
43. 1 Bottle of 500 Multi-Vitamins
44. 8 Cans of Tuna
45. 50 Pounds of Wheat
46. 6 Pounds of Macaroni
47. 20 Pounds of Sugar

48. 5 Cans of Cream of Mushroom Soup
49. 5 Pounds of Honey
50. 20 Pounds of Sugar
51. 8 Cans of Tomato Soup
52. 50 Pounds of Wheat

At the completion of one year of shopping, you would have amassed the following:

- 500 Pounds of Wheat
- 100 Pounds of Sugar
- 40 Pounds of Powdered Milk
- 12 Pounds of Salt
- 10 Pounds of Honey
- 5 Pounds of Peanut Butter
- 45 Cans of Tomato Soup
- 15 Cans of Cream of Mushroom Soup
- 24 Cans of Tuna
- 15 Cans of Cream of Chicken Soup
- 21 Boxes of Macaroni and Cheese
- 500 Aspirin
- 1,000 Multi-Vitamins
- 6 Pounds of Yeast
- 6 Pounds of Shortening
- 12 Pounds of Macaroni

This equals a diet of 2,000 calories a day for ten months for two people. While this is not a full year supply, you would not starve if you supplement it with foraging and some level of food production.

This technique has been widely circulated in preparedness circles over the years because it works. Even if you don't follow this particular list, spending a regular structured amount is the best way to get started in building a good food pantry.

Project 1:

Identifying and Procuring Food Grade Buckets for Storage

Whether you are just starting out storing food or are an experienced preparedness guru, you will need buckets to store all your food. When you are just starting out, buckets seem to be hard to find, but soon you will be swimming in them.

The easiest way to acquire buckets is to purchase them, but I have had great luck getting them from restaurants. They are also available for purchase from various stores.

The issue with using buckets for storing food is that you both have to ensure that the bucket was created to a "food grade" standard, and that it was never used to store anything that was not food grade.

The term food grade comes from US Food and Drug Administration (FDA) regulations.

The FDA requires that plastic used to package food should not contain dyes or recycled plastic that is deemed harmful to humans. Not only that—the mold release agents are also different.

To keep up with the various standards and regulations, the Society of Plastics Industry has established a seven-point system of labeling food-grade plastics. On each plastic container (normally on the bottom), there is a triangle-shaped label with rounded corners made of three arrows. The number in the center of the arrows identifies the type of plastic used in the container.

Below are the various types, symbols, and normal applications:

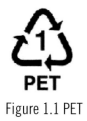

Figure 1.1 PET

PET or PETE (polyethylene terephthalate) is clear, tough, and has good gas and moisture barrier properties. This resin is commonly used in beverage bottles and many injection-molded consumer product containers. This plastic is normally called polyester.

HDPE

Figure 1.2 HDPE

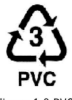

PVC

Figure 1.3 PVC

LDPE

Figure 1.4 LDPE

PP

Figure 1.5 PP

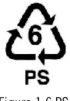

PS

Figure 1.6 PS

HDPE (high density polyethylene) is used in milk, juice, and water containers in order to take advantage of its protective barrier properties. Its chemical resistance properties also make it well suited for items such as containers for household chemicals and detergents. Most five-gallon food buckets are made from HDPE. Most (but not all) food grade buckets are type 2 HDPE. However, due to mold release agents and manufacturing processes, unless your #2 bucket is specifically labeled "food safe," assume that it is not.

Vinyl (polyvinyl chloride, or PVC) provides excellent clarity, puncture resistance and cling. When used as a film, PVC can breathe enough to be ideal for packaging fresh meats that require oxygen to ensure a bright red surface, while still protecting the food from contamination. 3 PVC is used to make plastic food wrap, shrink wrap, garden hoses, and shoe soles.

LDPE (low density polyethylene) offers clarity and flexibility. It is used to make bottles that require flexibility, such as squeeze bottles. Because of its strength and toughness, it is used as a film to make grocery bags and garbage bags, shrink and stretch film, and coating for milk cartons.

PP (polypropylene) has high tensile strength, making it ideal for use in caps and lids that have to hold tightly onto threaded openings. Because of its high melting point, polypropylene can be hot-filled with products designed to cool in bottles, including ketchup and syrup.

It is also used for products that need to be incubated, such as yogurt.

PS (polystyrene) is a colorless plastic that can be clear and hard. Additionally it can also be foamed to provide exceptional insulation properties. Foamed or expanded polystyrene (EPS) is used for products such as meat trays, egg cartons, and coffee cups. It is also used for packaging and protecting appliances, electronics, and other sensitive products.

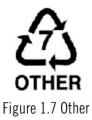

OTHER

Figure 1.7 Other

Other: This category basically means "everything else" and is composed of plastics that were invented after 1987. Plastics labeled as grade 7 should be specifically noted as being "food safe" before they are used to package or handle food.

For the home processor of stored food, types 2, 4, and 5 plastics are your safest bets as food safe buckets, as some type 1 plastics contain Bisphenol A which can interfere with human hormonal messaging. Additionally, as mentioned before, plastic that is marked food grade may still introduce unsafe contaminants due to its usage or manufacturing processes.

There are three ways to be sure that your buckets and barrels are truly "food safe":

1. Purchase new buckets that are marked "food grade" by the manufacturer. Often, the barrels will additionally be marked with "NSF," "FDA," or "USDA Approved."
2. Salvage used buckets that have already been used to store food and haven't been used for anything else. I have had good results getting food grade buckets for free from local delis (even if the buckets smelled strongly of the pickles that were their former occupants).
3. Call the manufacturer and ask.

Note: If a food grade bucket has been used to store non-food items like chemicals, paint, or detergent, it is no longer food grade.

When I get pickle buckets from my local deli, I wash the buckets with soap and water, follow that up with a bleach rinse, and air them out for a couple of days in the sun. If the bucket still smells, I dump in two cups or so of baking soda (the stronger the vinegar smell, the more I use), press on the lid, and let sit for a couple more days. After rinsing it out, the barrel should be nice and deodorized.

Project 2: Storing Food With Dry Ice

This project is an alternative method to help preserve your food storage. It is slightly more complicated than using oxygen absorbers, but it is cheaper. Additionally, depending on your location, this method is easier to do since most large grocery stores, as well as welding supply companies, stock dry ice. On the other hand, oxygen absorbers usually have to be ordered online.

In case you do not know, dry ice is just frozen carbon dioxide gas—as a block of CO_2 warms to room temperature, it turns into a harmless gas. Since one pound of the ice will turn into almost 8 ½ cubic feet of gas, it does not take much to fill the air spaces around your tiny grains of rice or wheat berries.

As a matter of fact, when using dry ice to replace the oxygen in your food storage buckets, the biggest risk is using too much, which could pop the top of your bucket.

The other hazards involved with dry ice are that it becomes a solid at 110°F below zero—so frostbite is likely if you handle it improperly—and that the CO_2 will displace the oxygen in the air (so do this outside or in a very well-ventilated room) so that you won't suffocate if you stick your head in a bucket of carbon dioxide. A good piece of information to keep in the back of your head is that PETA and other animal "rights" groups find suffocation by CO_2 to be the most humane way of dispatching small livestock (such as chickens)—for example, putting them in a bucket with a little CO_2 will suffocate them quickly. Personally, I disagree and could think of better ways to die than being stuck in a confined space and having all my air sucked out of my room, but what do I know . . .

Actually, dry ice can be a lot of fun. Put a cube in a glass of water and kids will enjoy watching the thick cloud that boils off. It will compete with your TV, at least for a while.

Remember when I said that a pound of solid carbon dioxide was about 8.5 cubic feet of gas? Well, 8.3 cubic feet is a closer measurement, and since a 6-gallon bucket is 1.46 cubic feet of space, a single pound of solid carbon dioxide would fill a lot of buckets. Add to that the food itself, which also takes up space. You will only need about .5 cubic foot of gas per 6-gallon bucket to fill about 80 buckets with 5 pounds of dry ice (at one ounce of solid CO_2 per bucket—which is actually a *lot* more than you need).

If you have some dry ice left, you can use it to do neat things like creating a fog if you drop it in water. If you drop some in a bowl of rubbing alcohol, you can get the alcohol cold enough to make a "poor man's dry ice."

The big thing to remember when using dry ice to purge out and replace the air in your bucket is that quality matters—if you get dry ice that has frozen water crystals on the block, then when the CO_2 melts, the water will be trapped at the bottom of your bucket. What you want to avoid is opening your wheat thirty years later to find that the water has combined with your food to make a nasty mold sludge instead of tasty wheat goodness. You can tell you have water crystals in your dry ice because dry ice is light blue and frozen water is white. So, when you bring your ice home, keep it in a plastic container with a tight (but not airtight) lid so that the constantly escaping CO_2 will push water away and let it form frost on your container instead of on your block.

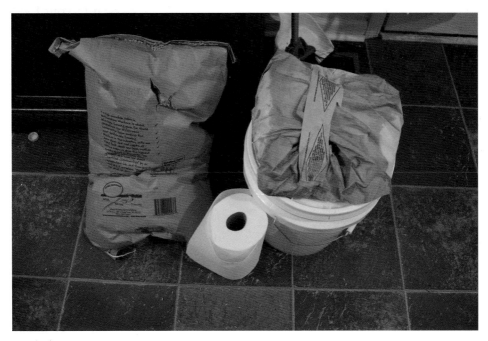

Figure 2.1 The ingredients

Materials:

- Bucket with tight-fitting lid
- Dry ice in plastic container (do not use glass or anything that will shatter under pressure, as you cannot keep the dry ice cold enough at your home to prevent it from turning back into gas)
- Hammer to break block
- Small scale to measure the weight of the dry ice chunks—you don't have to be exact in your measurements, but you need to be pretty close.
- Gloves (unless you want frostbite, do not handle ice with bare skin)
- Food to be stored

Procedure:

1. Break your ice into small chunks (one ounce by weight will be about ⅙ cup by volume, approximately).

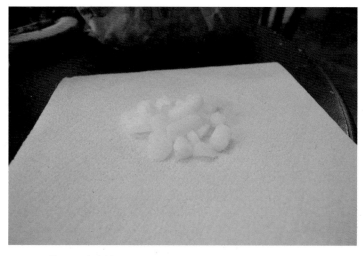

Figure 2.2 Use pellets or break into small chunks.

2. Pour one ounce (or two if you feel generous) into the bottom of your bucket and mound in a small pile in the center of your container.

3. Cover pile with a paper towel to keep your dry ice away from your food (not strictly necessary, but it makes my wife feel better).

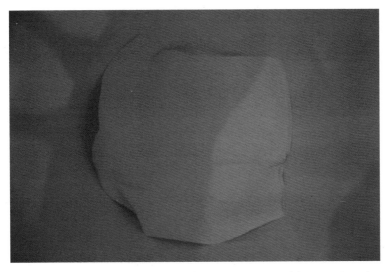

Figure 2.3 Pour into bottom of bucket and cover with paper towel.

4. Fill bucket with food to ½ inch of head space from top of bucket.

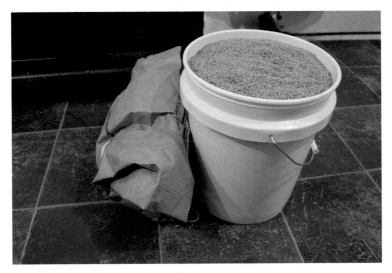

Figure 2.4 Fill to ½ inch from top of bucket.

5. Set the lid lightly on top and wait for ice to melt (if you seal the lid the expanding gas will "explode" the bucket—probably just popping the lid, but also possibly spewing food throughout your house especially if you are sealing powders like flour). You can seal the lid all the way around, except for a tiny gap on one side.

6. To tell when the dry ice has evaporated, feel the bottom of the bucket. If it is ice cold, you still have solid CO_2. It should take a day or so for the ice to totally dissipate.

7. As soon as the ice has turned to gas, seal the lid completely

8. Wait about 15 minutes and carefully check your buckets for signs of gas pressure. If the lids or sides of the bucket are bulged, then you still had dry ice in the bucket and need to crack the seal carefully. Check again after 10 minutes.

9. After the bucket is sealed, a vacuum may be present in your bucket and the sides may suck in a bit. This is normal and can be a good thing as no bugs will survive in a vacuum for long.

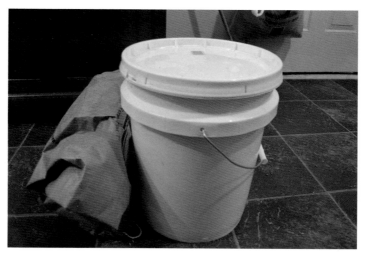

Figure 2.5 Sealed bucket of wheat

Yield:

Five pounds of ice (normally the minimum purchase) will do 40 buckets at 2 ounces per bucket, or 80 buckets at the necessary one ounce per 6-gallon bucket.

Note:

This is not a project in which you can buy the materials and do it later—the ice will dissipate into CO_2 even if stored in your deep freezer. If you buy dry ice, plan on using it within 5 or 6 hours.

Project 3: Coroplast to Vacuum Seal Mylar

No matter the brand, consumer vacuum sealers are not designed to work with Mylar bags. The inside of Mylar bags are smooth, whereas the insides of the plastic bags designed for use with vacuum sealers have ridges that allow air to freely flow out of the bag with the sides pressed together.

After much research into clamps, homemade vacuum chambers, and lots of trial and error, it was discovered that a strip of corrugated plastic called coroplast can be used to create a channel that will allow the vacuum sealer to evacuate the air out of the bag.

Coroplast is most often associated with political yard signs and is very easy to recycle.

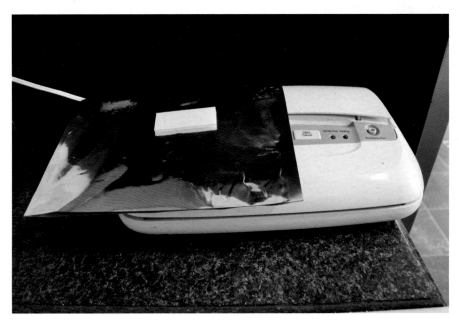

Figure 3.1 The equipment

Equipment:

- Mylar Bag (I prefer 7 mil one-gallon bags.)
- Foodsaver™ or any other consumer vacuum sealer
- Strip of coroplast (approximately 1 inch x 3 inch)—ensure that the corrugated strips run lengthways.
- Mylar Impulse sealer or iron and small board as long as the bag is wide.

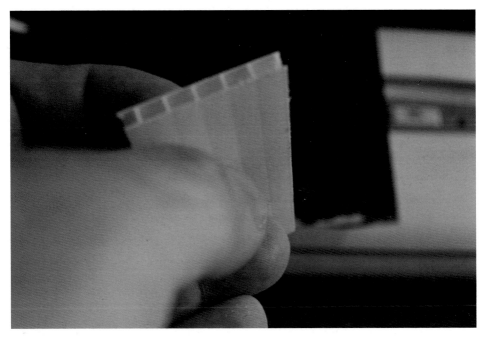

Figure 3.2 Lengthways, not widthways

Procedure:

1. Fill your Mylar bag with food (or ammo or spare parts). Leave room for the sealer to close around the mouth of the bag.

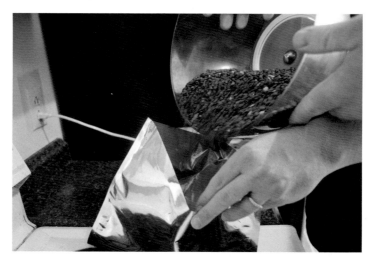

Figure 3.3 Fill the bag.

2. Insert the strip of coroplast into the bag, ensuring that one end is past the seal and into the vacuum chamber.

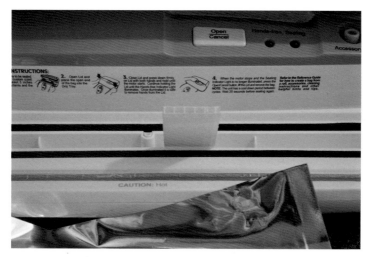

Figure 3.4 Strip must fit into the vacuum chamber of the sealer.

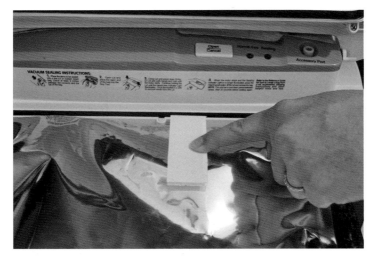

Figure 3.5 Strip must also fit past the seal of the machine.

3. Activate the machine. In the model I have, you press down on the lid until a light comes on, indicating a good vacuum has been achieved.

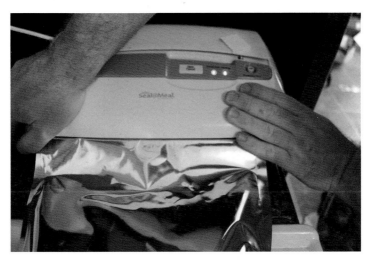

Figure 3.6 You should see the air being removed from the bag.

4. The internal sealer is not strong enough to make a reliable seal with a thick Mylar bag. You will either need to use an impulse sealer between the machine and the stored items in the bag, or you can place a board under the bag and seal it with an iron on medium heat.

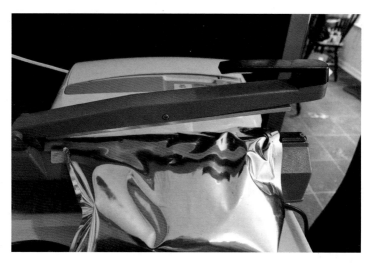

Figure 3.7 Use a secondary sealer to ensure a strong seal.

Note:
Depending on your machine and the bags you use, you may need to experiment with the optimal placement of the coroplast strip. It took some fiddling until I could get a consistent seal.

Project 4: Oven Canning

You will never find this technique in a USDA or National Center for Home Preservation website; there are just too many variables to say that the process works 100 percent every time with every food type.

However, if you reread the section on food safety, you will see that botulism needs moisture as well as anaerobic conditions to grow. That means that the only items you should oven can should be dried. This makes it really good for items like pancake mix or flour.

This process should not be used with wheat berries or anything you plan on sprouting as the temperatures will most likely kill them. Luckily, the process will kill any mealworms or other insects that tend to infest (in allowable levels according to FDA standards) wheat or flour process.

What happens is the heat kills any live infestations, and as the air expands with the heat, it is pushed out of the jar. So as it cools, the lids will seal, creating a good vacuum seal, which prevents any moisture or bacteria from entering.

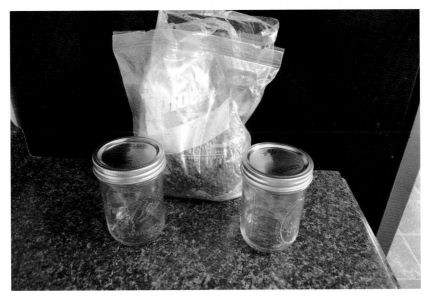

Figure 4.1 The ingredients

Equipment:

- Canning jars
- Canning lids and screw bands
- Wide mouth funnel
- Dried goods

  - White rice, oats, and other grains
  - Beans and lentils
  - Flour
  - Baking mixes
  - Spices, salt, baking soda, etc.

- Oven
- Pot holders and towels

Procedure:

1. Preheat oven to 200°F.
2. Fill your sterile canning jars with dried goods, leaving ½ inch head space. Do not put lids on yet.
3. Place in oven and heat for one hour.

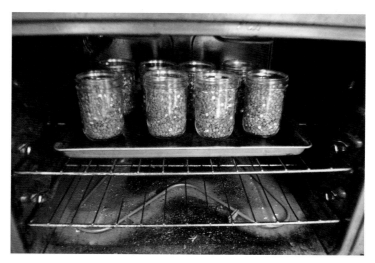

Figure 4.2 Heat without lids first.

4. Use pot holders or towel to remove jars from oven.
5. Quickly wipe rim of jar with damp (but not dripping) towel.

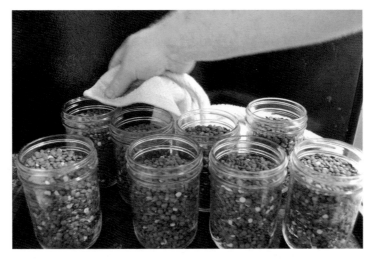

Figure 4.3 Wipe lids with damp towel.

6. Place metal canning lid on jar and screw metal band on tightly.
7. Return jars to oven and set timer for 30 minutes.
8. Remove jars from oven and allow to cool.

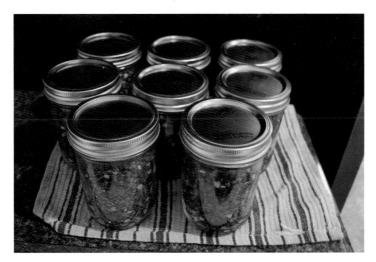

Figure 4.4 Let cool.

9. Check lids for tight seal.

Yield:

Variable

Notes:

Do not use plastic canning lids.

Oven canning is not a safe method of preserving anything other than dried goods. Do *not* use this method for canning wet foods such as fruits, vegetables, or meats unless they have been thoroughly dehydrated. Be sure to label your jars with the contents, date canned, and how to prepare.

Once your jars of dried goods have cooled and you have checked the seal to ensure that it "popped," store them in a cool, dark, and dry location. The seal will prevent moisture from getting into the jars, but moist air will rust metal canning lids and bands.

Whole grains store better than grains that have been ground into meal or flour.

If you are canning baking mixes, ensure that they do not contain shortening (it will melt), oil (will turn rancid), or brown sugar (has moisture).

Project 5:
Butter from Powdered Milk

This recipe is a common food storage technique as butter can be hard to store. Additionally, those who store 16 pounds or more of powdered milk per person per year (double or triple for homes with children), following the plan attributed to the Church of Latter Day Saints, need recipes that use powdered milk.

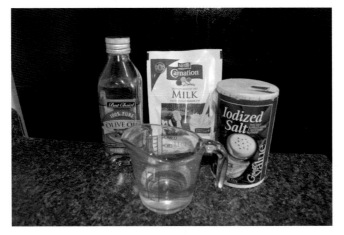

Figure 5.1 The ingredients

Ingredients:

- ¾ cup powdered milk
- ⅓ cup water
- ¼ cup oil (coconut, olive, or sunflower)

Alternatively, you can use yellow food coloring, salt, or butter flavoring—but I only use a pinch of salt.

Equipment:

- Blender (I like using my mason jar on the blender, as I can store the butter directly in the jar.)
- Measuring cup

Procedure:

1. Add the powdered milk to your food processor, blender jar, or bowl.

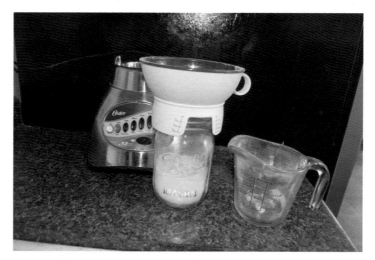

Figure 5.2 A canning funnel cuts down on mess.

2. Add ⅓ cup of water.

3. Add ¼ cup of oil—I used olive oil, but almost any kind of oil will do in a pinch.

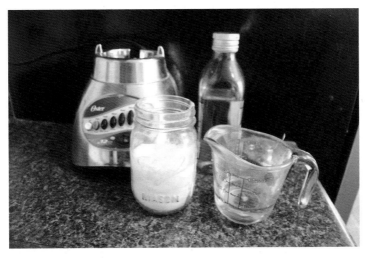

Figure 5.3 Oil is necessary for the buttery consistency.

4. Blend for a few quick pulses. Check often to check for thickening. Keep blending until it starts getting thick. In my experience, it does not take long at all.

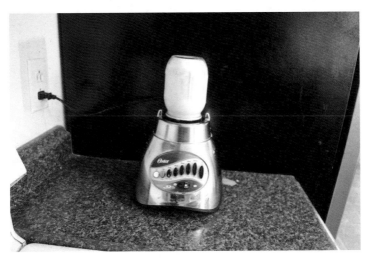

Figure 5.4 I prefer to use a mason jar, but make sure you tighten it down well or it may leak.

5. If you want a yellow color, salted butter, or a more buttery flavor, you can now mix in the butter flavoring, yellow coloring, and/or salt (optional).

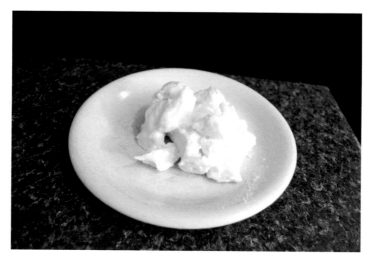

Figure 5.5 The finished butter should have a smooth look of margarine.

Yield:

Approximately ¾ cup or one "stick"

Note:

The taste was similar to butter, and the texture was right, but this may not be a good choice for sautéing—it browned and crumbled when I used it to make a butter sauce (it tasted fine, and the texture was not bad; it was just unexpected).

Project 6: Cream-of-Whatever Soup

Typical canned food bought in bulk at Aldi or warehouse stores makes up a significant portion of my family's food storage plan. It is simple, lasts several years, and fits like a glove in the "store what you eat, eat what you store" philosophy.

However, as easy as it is to use canned soups as bases for recipes, it is not the most frugal way of doing things. Here, I will show you how to make a simple base for cream-of-whatever soup. If you want cream of chicken use chicken stock, or for tomato use tomato juice—it's that simple . . .

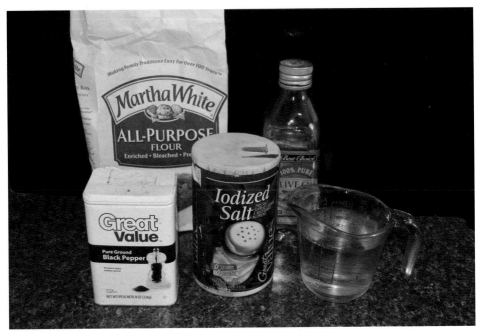

Figure 6.1 The ingredients

Ingredients:

- 3 tablespoons butter or oil
- 3 tablespoons flour
- ¼ teaspoon salt
- Dash of pepper
- 1 ¼ cups liquid, milk or stock

Equipment:

- Saucepan
- Measuring cup
- Spoon
- Wire whisk

Procedure:

1. Melt butter or oil in saucepan.

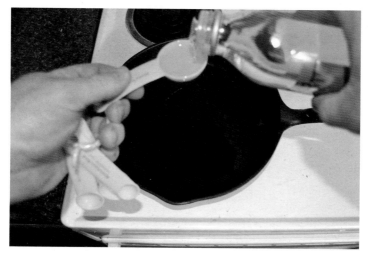

Figure 6.2 Add fats.

2. Stir in flour.

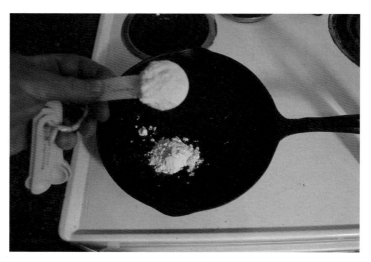

Figure 6.3 Add flour.

3. Add spices.

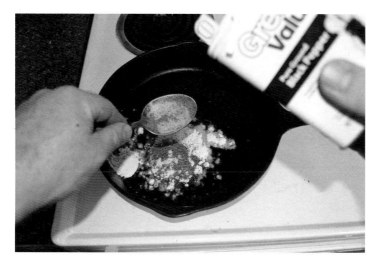

Figure 6.4 Add salt, pepper, and any spices to taste.

4. Cook over medium heat until oil and flour are fully incorporated.

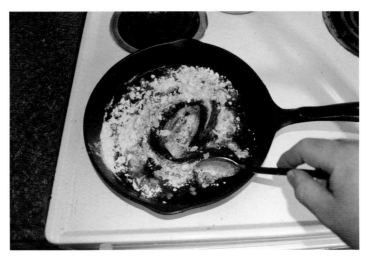

Figure 6.5 Mix and cook well.

5. Add liquid slowly, stirring with wire whisk to prevent lumps.

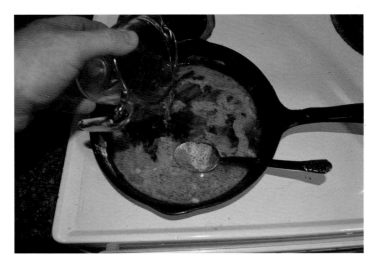

Figure 6.6 The liquid added determines type of soup.

6. Cook until thick.

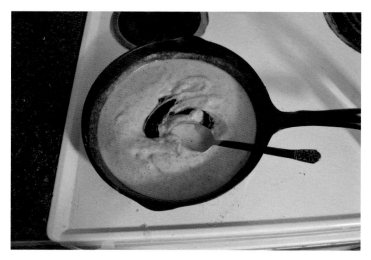

Figure 6.7 Cook until thick.

Yield:
Makes the equivalent to 1 can of condensed soup.

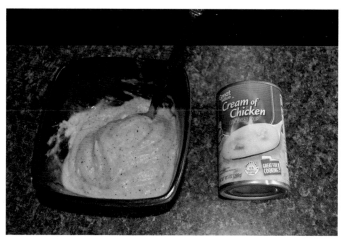

Figure 6.8 It's much cheaper than canned soup.

Variations:

This is a very versatile mix that is only limited by your imagination.

Tomato Soup: Use tomato juice for the liquid. Add dashes of garlic, onion powder, basil, and oregano.

Chicken Soup: Use chicken broth for half the liquid. Add ¼ teaspoon of poultry seasoning or sage.

Mushroom/celery/chive soup: Sauté ¼ cup chopped mushrooms, celery, or chives and 1 tablespoon minced onion in butter before adding flour.

Allergy Suggestion:

If you use a gluten-free flour (rice, tapioca, etc.) or cornstarch, you can make the soup gluten-free. And if you use a stock rather than milk, you can make it milk-free, too.

Project 7: Emergency Baby Formula

Obviously, human breast milk is the perfect food for infants. However, there are a variety of instances that could make breast milk unavailable during a catastrophic disaster.

You may think: why can't I just give my child cow's milk? Well, about 40 percent of normal infants cannot tolerate cow's milk and may have intestinal blood loss. Cow's milk also does not have enough iron, and it has too much protein (which taxes a baby's kidneys).

Today's project provides a workable emergency substitute.

I encourage you to speak with your pediatrician about these recipes before trying them with your children, as I am neither a doctor, nor am I familiar with the constitution of your baby.

Also, it is important to note that these recipes are for *emergency* substitutions and are not designed to be used long term.

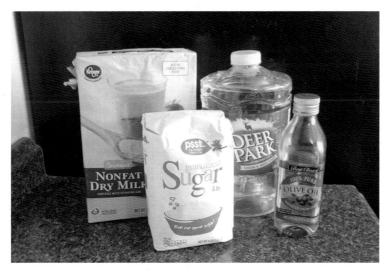

Figure 7.1 The ingredients

Ingredients:

- ⅓ cup plus 2 tablespoons of instant powdered milk
- 1 ½ cup boiled water
- 1 tablespoon oil
- 2 teaspoons sugar

Equipment:

- Measuring cup
- Spoon
- Funnel
- Baby bottle

Procedure:

1. Mix powdered milk and water.

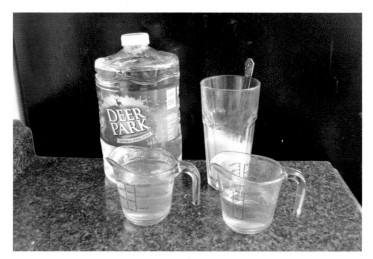

Figure 7.2 Mix sterile water and powdered milk.

2. Blend thoroughly.

3. Add oil and sugar.

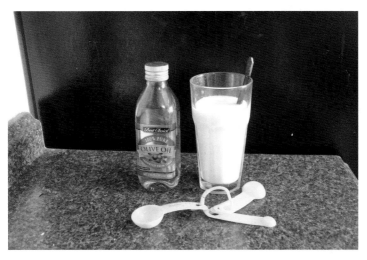

Figure 7.3 Mix oil and sugar.

4. Add to baby bottle.

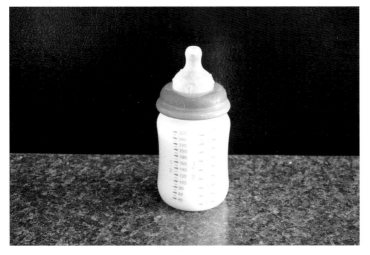

Figure 7.4 Put in a bottle.

Yield:
　　2 bottles (3 if newborn)

Project 8: Magic Mix

This is another recipe that is very well known to the prepping community. It makes great use of stored dry milk, and it makes family cooking much easier and cheaper as it is the base for many common convenience food mixes.

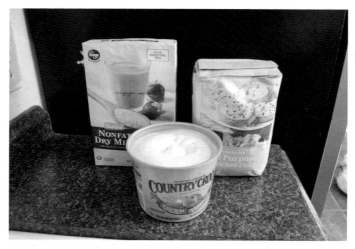

Figure 8.1 The ingredients

Ingredients:

- 2 ⅓ cup non-instant powdered milk instant powdered milk
- 1 cup all-purpose flour
- 1 cup real margarine (not spread) or butter, at room temperature

Equipment:

- Bowl
- Measuring cup
- Mason jar/lid

Preparation:

1. Combine dry milk, flour, and margarine/butter in a large bowl.

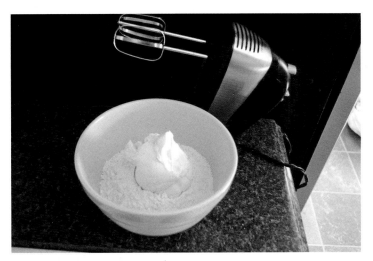

Figure 8.2 Combine ingredients.

2. Mix with electric mixer until it looks like cornmeal (this can take a while as you want to break it up into very small bits).

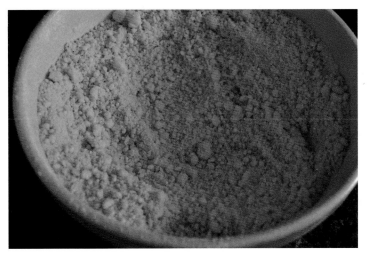

Figure 8.3 Mix until thoroughly combined.

3. Keep mix tightly covered in the refrigerator. It will stay good up to 2 months.
4. If you do not have butter or margarine, you can also use the following recipe to get a similar mix that can be substituted for most magic mix recipes:

Alternative Preparation:

- 4 cups instant nonfat dry milk
- 1 cup flour
- ½ cup vegetable oil

Follow the same procedure as original mix.

Yield:
4 ⅓ cups original mix or 5 ½ cups using the alternative recipe

Note:
This can be used in all manner of recipes, with the cheese sauce below being one of my favorites.

Magic Cheese Dip

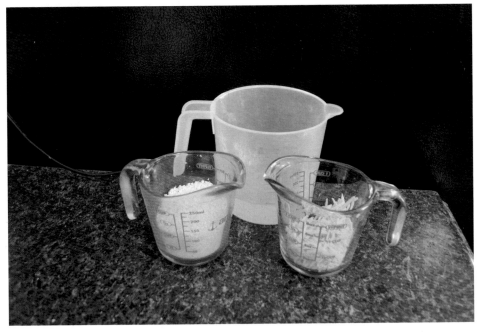

Figure 8.4 Cheese mix ingredients

Ingredients:

- ½–⅔ cup Magic Mix (depending on desired thickness)
- 1 cup water
- ¼ cup grated cheddar cheese

Equipment:

- Measuring cup
- Saucepan
- Spoon

Procedure:

1. Heat water and Magic Mix in a saucepan over low/medium heat until smooth and creamy.
2. Add cheese and stir constantly until melted and fully mixed.

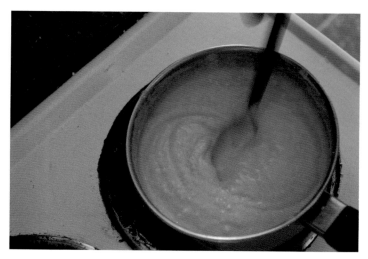

Figure 8.5 Heat and mix until smooth.

Project 9:
Emergency Food Bar

Emergency food needs to be shelf stable and to contain necessary nutrients. It is a plus if the food tastes good, is light weight, and not very expensive. This is not the easiest project to achieve, and I had to test many different recipes until I settled on this one.

This particular food bar recipe produces a hard biscuit that is reminiscent of both hardtack and the commercial Datrex bar. It is not a gourmet meal, but it is light and, if stored properly, can last for well over a year.

This is a very simple recipe, and the base recipe I used can be found on many websites. I found that by modifying the recipe and making small "cakes" instead of the more common loaf, I can make the food bar much easier to eat and handle.

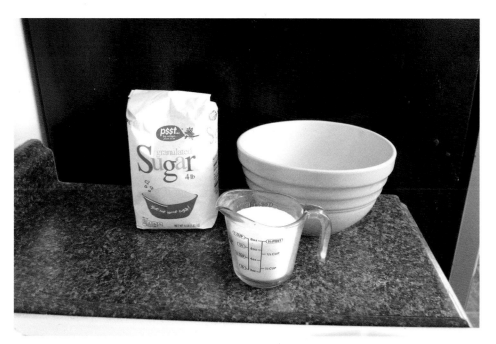

Figure 9.1 The ingredients

Ingredients:

- 2 cups oats (quick or flaked oats work equally well)
- 2 ½ cups powdered milk
- 1 cup sugar
- 3 tablespoons honey
- 1 3-oz package Jell-O (orange or lemon)
- 3 tablespoons water

Equipment:

- Bowl
- Measuring cup
- Spoon
- Saucepan
- Parchment paper
- Cookie sheet
- Aluminum foil or plastic bag

Procedure:

1. Mix the oats, powdered milk, and sugar together in a bowl.

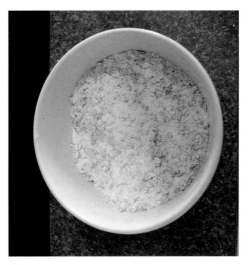

Figure 9.2 Mix dry ingredients.

2. In a medium pan mix 3 tablespoons of water, one package of Jell-O and 3 tablespoons of honey. Bring to a rolling boil. Due to the small amount of water and the high amount of sugar, this recipe is very sweet. If you use flavors other than lemon or orange you may find this bar to be *too* sweet.

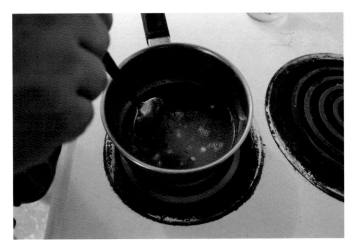

Figure 9.3 Bring Jell-O/water mix to a rolling boil.

3. Add Jell-O mixture to dry ingredients. Mix well. If the dough is too dry, add a small amount of water a teaspoon at a time. Do not use too much water because this bar only works if it is bone dry. The mixing process involves work. Mixers aren't strong enough and you will have to use your hands and arms.

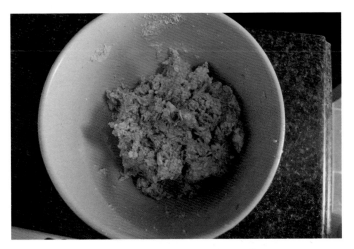

Figure 9.4 Mix wet and dry ingredients.

4. Preheat oven to 350°F.
5. Most food bar recipes will ask you to shape the well-mixed dough into loaves at this point. I found that by rolling the dough into ping pong–sized balls and smashing them into flat disks, the end product is much handier and easier to eat.

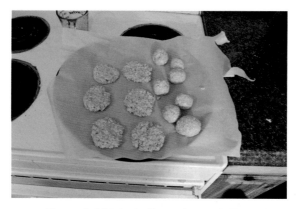

Figure 9.5 Make balls and smash flat.

6. Bake your bars at 350°F for 10–15 minutes. (If you are making a loaf, the time is more like 20 minutes.) You are not trying to cook the bar, but rather dry it out. I find that by propping the oven door open slightly, you will get a dryer bar (the dryer the bar, the safer you are from food-borne illnesses like botulism—and the bar will store longer). Alternatively, you may want to cook for 10 minutes and then place it in a dehydrator until completely dry.

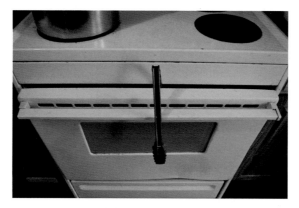

Figure 9.6 Prop oven door open.

7. Let cool completely.
8. Wrap in aluminum foil to store. Another benefit of the disk shape is that they can be rolled like coins. If you want to store these in your car or bug-out bag it would be a good idea to seal these in a vacuum bag after you put them in aluminum foil.

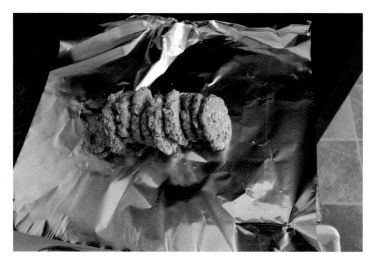

Figure 9.7 Wrap in aluminum foil.

Yield:
　This recipe equals approximately 2,000 calories, which is the suggested daily caloric intake for an average adult.

Project 10:
Canning Whole Grapes

This project made it into the book for several reasons. It is a very novel and easy introduction to water bath canning. Secondly, it's a great way to store grapes. Lastly, depending on the sugar used, it makes an awesome grape juice *or* juice concentrate.

Since we photographed this in the winter, we used two average bags of grapes from the grocery store and the yield changed accordingly, but an average of 14 pounds is needed per canner load of 7 quarts. If you are canning in pints, you can expect one pound per pint. If you are buying from a farmer, a lug of grapes is 26 pounds.

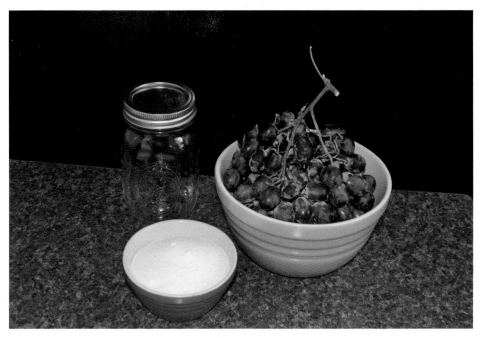

Figure 10.1 The ingredients

Ingredients:

- Slightly unripe, tight-skinned, green seedless grapes are preferred, but I have used store-bought purple grapes without any problems.
- Sugar*
- Water*
  *Amounts of sugar and water depend on types of canning syrup desired. There is a chart below with specific amounts and ratios.

Equipment:

- Measuring cup
- Pot
- Canning funnel
- Sterile canning jars, lids, and rings
- Water bath canner
- Canning jar lifter
- Towel

Procedure:

1. Stem, wash, and drain grapes.

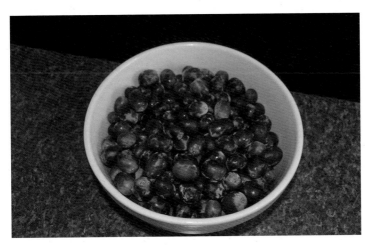

Figure 10.2 If you have a helper to stem grapes, buy extra just in case they get eaten . . .

2. Fill your water bath canner with water to a level that is approximately 1 inch over the top of the jar and begin heating water to a boil.
3. Prepare syrup by mixing water and sugar, and heating to a boil.

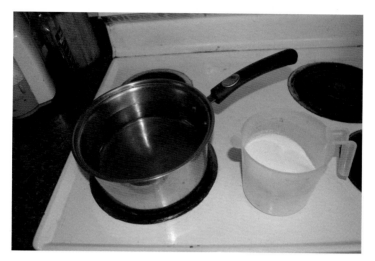

Figure 10.3 Mixing syrup

Mixture of water and sugar					
		9 pint load		7 quart load	
Syrup Type	Approximate % Sugar	Cups Water	Cups Sugar	Cups Water	Cups Sugar
Very Light	10	6 ½	¾	10 ½	1 ¼
Light	20	5 ¾	1 ½	9	2 ¼
Medium	30	5 ¼	2 ¼	8 ¼	3 ¾
Heavy	40	5	3 ¼	7 ¾	5 ¼
Very Heavy	50	4 ¼	4 ¼	6 ½	6 ¾

4. In my experience, very light or light syrup makes a juice that you can drink straight from the jar, but heavy or very heavy syrup needs diluting.

5. Raw pack by filling jars with grapes.

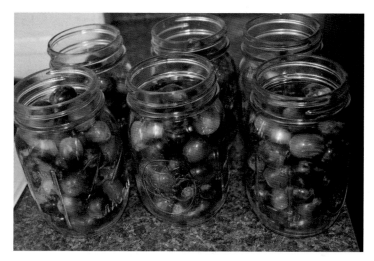

Figure 10.4 After eating many of my grapes, I had to supplement the recipe with a few white grapes.

6. Add hot syrup, leaving 1 inch of head space from top of the jar.

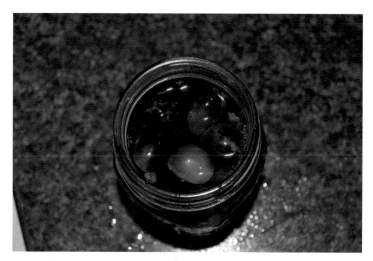

Figure 10.5 Leave one inch of space between top of jar and top of liquid.

7. Wipe the tops of the jars with a towel.
8. Place sterilized rings and lids on your jars and tighten slightly.
9. Place filled jars in the boiling water of your canner using your canning jar lifter, and process.
10. Pints need to boil for 20 minutes. Quarts need to boil for 25 minutes.

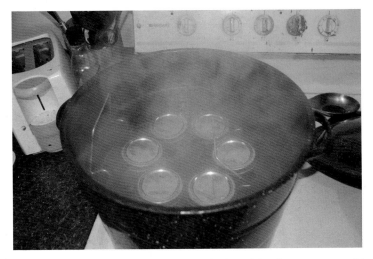

Figure 10.6 If the water stops boiling during this phase, you need to bring the water back to a boil and restart the clock.

Yield:

Depending on amounts of fruit used, the yield will vary. Typically, to reduce energy waste, only full canner loads of 7 quarts or 9 pints are done at a time.

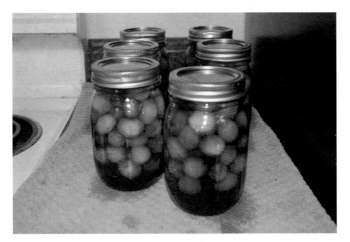

Figure 10.7 Finished grapes

Notes:

Fruits may also be canned in water or fruit juice instead of using syrup. The syrup does not preserve the fruit but it does help maintain the shape, color, and flavor of your grapes.

Unsweetened apple juice, pineapple juice, and white grape juice also make good canning liquids. These may be used directly or diluted with water.

Additionally, mild-flavored honey may be used to replace up to half the table sugar called for in syrups.

Do not use artificial sweeteners as saccharin-based sweeteners can become bitter and aspartame-based sweeteners may lose their sweetening power during processing.

Project 11: Brandied Fruit

This is a great way to preserve fresh fruit without having to deal with the heat of canning, making it perfect for the summer.

We have brandied several fruits, from strawberries to apples. Our experience with apples is that even after a year the apples are just as crisp as they were when we first brandied them. However, the apples have absorbed the majority of the alcohol and they taste more like alcohol than apple. Depending on your tastes and uses, this can either be a good or a bad thing.

Strawberries break down and are better suited to use as a strawberry shortcake topping (they make a very good dumpcake* base).

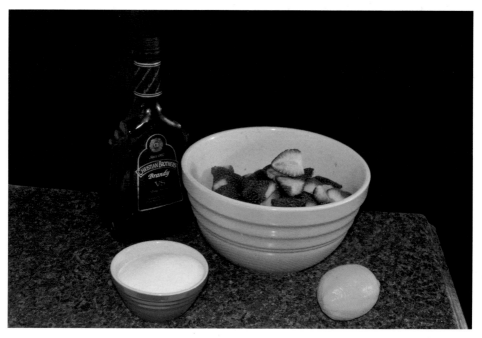

Figure 11.1 The ingredients

Ingredients:

- 1 cup fruit (sliced)
- 2 cups water
- 1 cup sugar
- 2 tablespoons lemon juice (This step is optional but it does two things: it helps reduce browning of the fruit and it inverts the sugar.**)
- 1 cup brandy (We have used white whiskey and vodka successfully, but brandy adds a nice taste.)

Equipment:

- Pot
- Spoon
- Measuring cup
- Canning funnel
- Sterile canning jars, lids, and rings

Procedure:

1. De-stem and slice your strawberries.

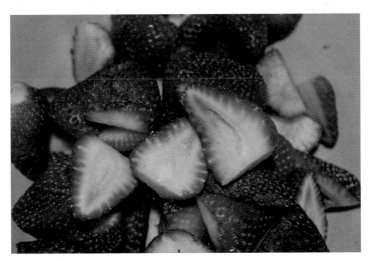

Figure 11.2 Sliced fruit

2. Mix water, sugar, and lemon juice in a pot and gently heat.
3. Add fruit and bring to a boil (do not leave the pot unattended, as the sugar can rapidly boil over).

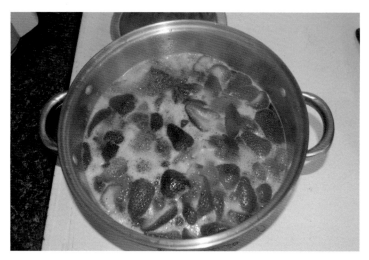

Figure 11.3 Do not leave boiling sugar syrup unattended.

4. Boil for 10 minutes while stirring occasionally.
5. Remove from heat and add any 80–120 proof alcohol.

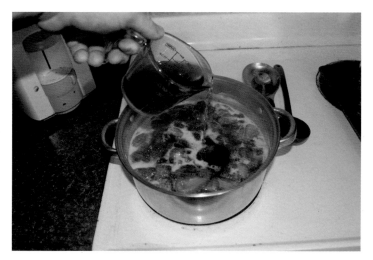

Figure 11.4 You may add more alcohol, but not less.

6. Use canning funnel to spoon mixture into sterile canning jars, leaving 1 inch of head space from the top of the jar.

7. Loosen rings and store for at least 2 weeks before using.

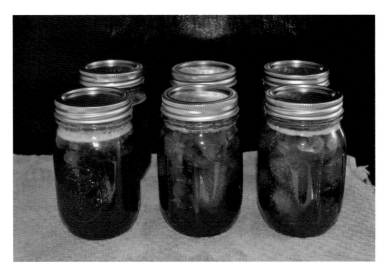

Figure 11.5 Our mixture yielded more syrup than fruit,
but the extra juice makes a great cordial base.

Yield:

This recipe can be increased proportionately. The amounts listed yield one pint.

Notes:

I have personal experience with storing high acid fruits in the refrigerator for two years with no negative results. As long as the alcohol covers the fruit and no additional moisture is added, the fruit should last indefinitely if stored appropriately.

*Dumpcake is made by dumping 2 pint jars of brandied fruit in a cake pan, covering it with dry cake mix, covering the mix with pats of butter, and baking for one hour in a 350°F oven.

** Inverted sugar is common in the processes of beekeeping and candy making. Sucrose (table sugar) is inverted by splitting it into glucose (grape sugar) and fructose (fruit sugar). Sugar is inverted by heating it in the presence of acid. Candy makers use inverted sugar to control crystallization and give candies extra moisture. Honey is very similar to inverted sugar, and beekeepers use it to feed bees if the keeper has harvested their entire winter honey store and taken it away to sell.

Project 12: Collecting Yeast

Yeast is a vital ingredient in many staple foods—without it bread won't rise, soda won't carbonate, and you cannot have either alcohol or vinegar to preserve food without yeast.

The problem is that local yeasts vary in quality. In order to get uniform results in your cooking/brewing, you either need to buy commercial yeasts or harvest a single batch of wild yeast and then cultivate it to use over and over.

The famous San Francisco sourdough is an example of this—the yeast cultures have been grown and reused over and over.

If you take care of your yeast it can live for hundreds of years.

The process is pretty simple, and it does not take a lot of effort to maintain for weekly bread making.

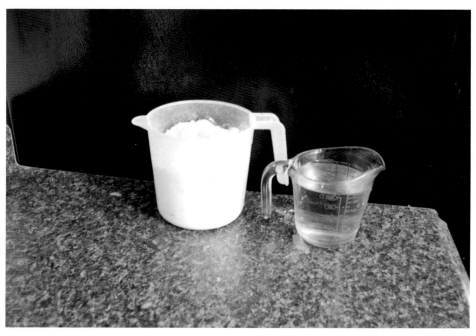

Figure 12.1 It only takes flour, water, and the natural yeast in the air.

Ingredients

- 3 cups water (distilled or boiled is best—I use tap water, but let it sit for a couple days to release the chlorine.)
- 3 cups all-purpose flour

Equipment:

- Measuring cup
- Mixing bowl
- Spoon
- Clean towel
- Quart mason jar and lid

Procedure:

1. Heat 2 cups of water to room temperature (about 85°F). The water needs to be as close to sterile as possible to prevent anything other than yeast to grow. The water also needs to be de-chlorinated—either by letting it sit for a couple days or by rapidly pouring it back or forth between two cups.
2. Mix together 2 cups of flour and 2 cups warm water. The mix does not have to be perfectly smooth. Some lumps are fine. However, the yeast you want floats in the air, so you need to mix vigorously to incorporate some air into the mix.

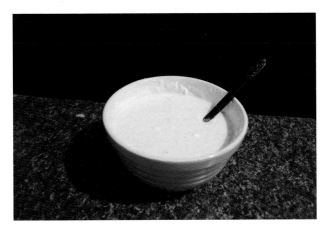

Figure 12.2 Mix well.

3. Cover your bowl lightly with a towel or a piece of cheesecloth. You do not want to use anything that will not allow air flow into the mix—so a plastic lid or wrap should not be used.

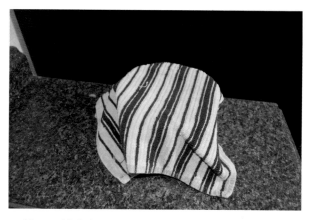

Figure 12.3 Cover with a towel, not plastic wrap.

4. Place the covered bowl in a warm protected area like inside a cold oven. Over the next day, stir every three or four hours to incorporate more air.

5. After 24 hours, check your starter and see if it has bubbles.

- If you do not see bubbles, whip the mix with a fork to incorporate more air and let sit for 24 more hours. (Depending on the quality of the wild yeast in your area this may take up to four days—it takes two at my house.)
- If you see a lot of bubbles then you have successfully collected yeast.

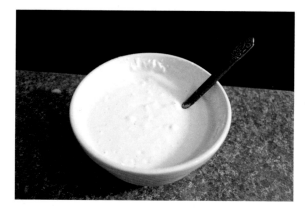

Figure 12.4 Bubbles mean success.

6. Add another cup of 85°F water and a cup of flour to feed your culture.

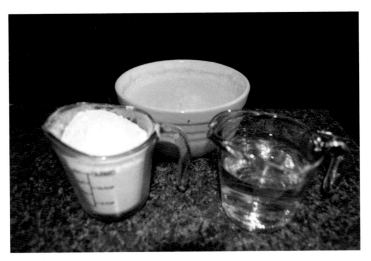

Figure 12.5 Feed the culture.

7. Store the mix in a quart mason jar with a loose lid.

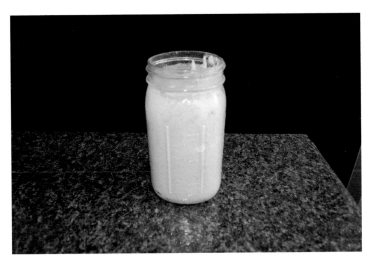

Figure 12.6 Store in a covered quart jar in the refrigerator.

Yield:

One cup of culture per loaf of bread is a good start—the exact ratios depend on the yeast and the desired loaf, so some experimentation is necessary.

Notes:

The culture will continue to be active at room temperature, so if you have a tight lid and keep the mix on your counter, the jar will explode.

The yeast will go inactive when cold, so for best results store in the refrigerator.

Every week, take out a cup of starter and replace with a cup of flour water mix—this feeds the yeast.

If you leave the culture alone for a few weeks, a liquid will separate and rise to the top. You can mix this back into the culture to bake with, but I have used this as a yeast to make wine (depending on the quality of your wild yeast, the taste of your wine may suffer or be improved).

Project 13: Dandelion Wine

Alcohol is quite useful even if you don't plan to drink it. It can be used to preserve food as alcohol, converted to vinegar for pickling, used medicinally, or bartered.

What is interesting is that wine can be made from almost any plant, as long as you have yeast and some form of sugar.

The neat thing about this recipe is that we are using something that is extremely common, easily harvested, and who many consider to be a weed. The best thing is that, while the greens are edible, the use of the flowers to make wine does not take food source off the table. Whenever I pick grapes or other fruit, I have to decide if I want to eat them or make alcohol from them. This isn't an issue with dandelions, as I am not going to eat the flowers.

Making wine is so easy that anyone can do it with just a small amount of equipment and knowledge.

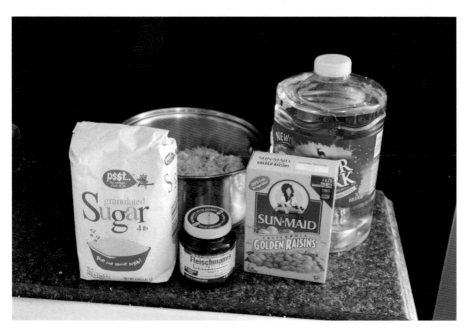

Figure 13.1 The ingredients

Ingredients:

- 1 quart of yellow dandelion flowers
- 8 cups of sugar
- 1 gallon of boiling water
- ¼ cup of raisins (to be used as yeast nutrient)
- 1 packet of yeast (it is possible to get away with wild yeast if you do not completely seal the fermentation container—but this is risky and you will probably end up with vinegar)
- 3 tablespoons (approximately) of vodka or other neutral spirit above 80 proof

Equipment:

- Saucepan
- Measuring cup
- Filtering bag or other straining equipment
- 1-gallon jug (I use old jugs from cheap table wine.)
- Bung and Airlock (Some use gloves or balloons with a small needle hole, but that is unreliable and a $2 dollar bung and airlock are much better solutions.)

Procedure:

1. Pick a quart of blossoms; you will be surprised at how small of a lawn it takes to get enough blossoms. Ideally, you should make the wine immediately after picking the flowers. However, you can freeze the flowers until you get enough.

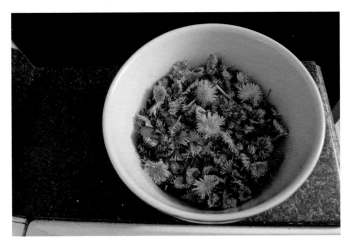

Figure 13.2 Bowl of flowers

2. Remove as much greenery from the blossoms as possible, as the sap from the stems will make the wine bitter over time. I find that you can pinch the base of the flower and press, allowing the yellow petals to "slide" out of the flower with little trouble.

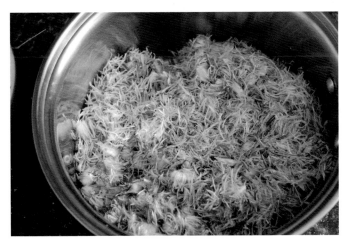

Figure 13.3 Flower petals

3. Boil the petals in one gallon of water for 5 minutes.

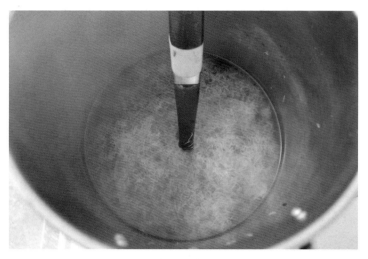

Figure 13.4 Boil petals.

4. Remove the blossoms, discard them, and let the water cool to about 90°F.

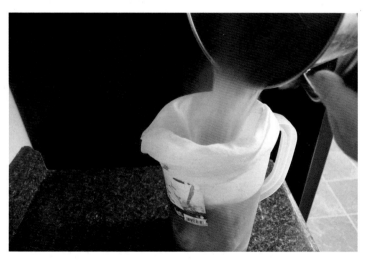

Figure 13.5 Filter out petals and let cool.

5. Add sugar to the warm juice.

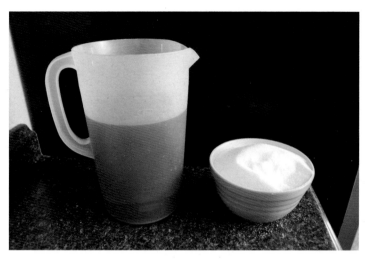

Figure 13.6 Add sugar.

6. Add a package of yeast. If you don't have wine yeast, a tablespoon of bread yeast will also work with good results.

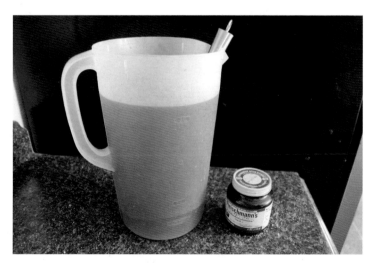

Figure 13.7 Add yeast.

7. Funnel the mix into a sterile container and add ¼ cup of raisins to feed the yeast.

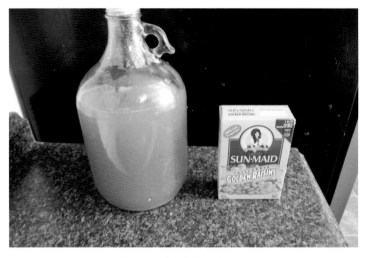

Figure 13.8 Add raisins.

8. Insert the bung into the top of the jug, insert the airlock into the top of the bung, and fill the airlock to the fill line with alcohol (the alcohol prevents mold or bacteria from growing in the airlock).

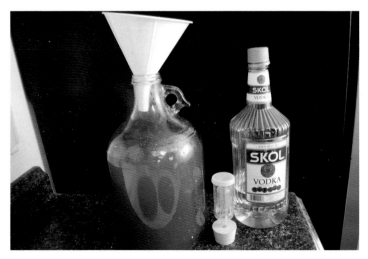

Figure 13.9 Add vodka to airlock.

9. Let the wine ferment for about 13 days. I usually put it in an unheated/uncooled closet. As long as you see bubbles in the airlock, the wine is fermenting.
10. Siphon your dandelion wine off the sediment in the fermentation container and seal it in jars. I have used mason jars, but wine bottles are much stronger.

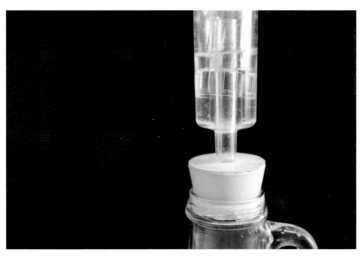

Figure 13.10 Airlock filled with alcohol

Project 14: Cardboard Box Grill

This project shows you an alternate cooking method that will allow you to bake or grill using a cardboard box. It's a simple little project, and only takes a few minutes to create out of very little material—which makes it much more portable than your grill.

Materials:

- 1 cardboard box with a slide-on top (like a banker box or a box that holds reams of paper)
- Heavy duty aluminum foil
- 1 pie plate (or other shallow metal container)
- 3 wire coat hangers
- Charcoal
- Matches
- White glue (optional)

Equipment:

- Scissors
- Pliers
- Tongs
- Sponge (optional)
- Food

Procedure:

1. Cut off the base of several coat hangers (I used 9), leave one bent end to form a "j" shape.

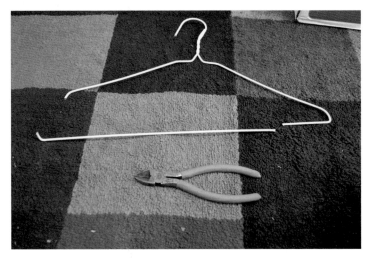

Figure 14.1 Cut coat hanger into a "j" shape.

2. If the coat hanger is plastic coated, strip off the coating. Sand if painted.
3. Line the inside of your box and lid with aluminum foil. If you want a sturdier oven, or if you are having a hard time keeping the foil in place, you can use a sponge to daub white glue or you can use a glue stick.

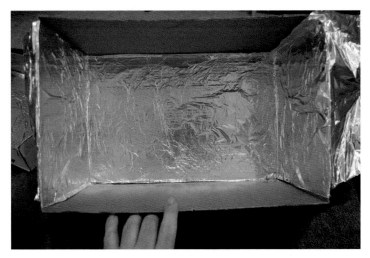

Figure 14.2 Line with aluminum foil.

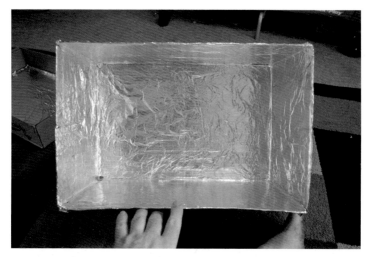

Figure 14.3 Ensure that the shiny side of the foil faces out.

4. Space your hangers equally along the side of your box—they will form a grill shelf.

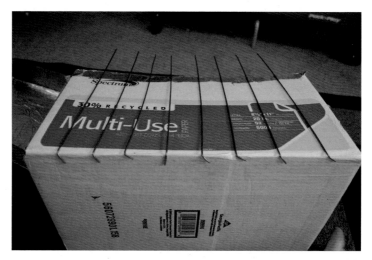

Figure 14.4 Space hangers equally.

5. Carefully push the hangers through the box side taking care not to rip the foil. Align the hangers on the opposite side of the box and punch them through the second wall of the box.

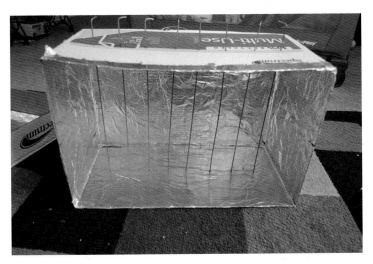

Figure 14.5 Form a shelf.

6. Bend your wires where they exit the box so they don't sag and allow food to fall into the coals.
7. Poke about 8–12 holes near the top of the box (evenly spaced on all four sides—2 or 3 per side). This lets gas out of the box.

8. Place some charcoals in the metal plate. To calculate heat in the paper box oven, you can figure that each charcoal briquette supplies 40°F of heat. This means you will need 9 briquettes to get a 360-degree oven.

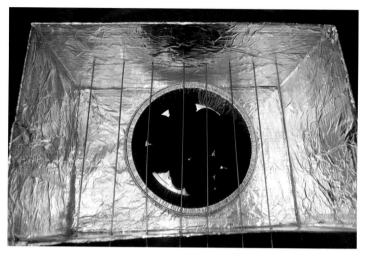

Figure 14.6 Put charcoal in pie plate.

9. Light your briquettes with matches or a lighter.
10. Let the briquettes burn for a while until they are all ignited and grey.
11. With your tongs, pick up the hot plate of charcoal and set it in the bottom of the box under the hanger wire shelf.
12. You want to arrange the charcoal evenly to get a consistent cooking temperature in the oven. If the charcoal is bunched, you will get hot spots.

13. Place your food on the wire racks.
14. Cover with your oven top.

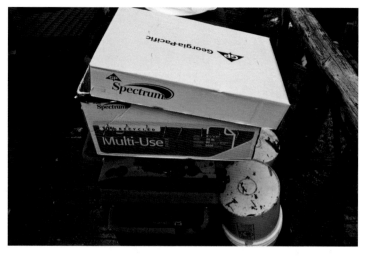

Figure 14.7 Put lid on and grill.

15. Bake as normal, but please note that after about 45 minutes the charcoal will start to burn out. As a result, for items with a longer cook time, you may need two pans of charcoal and switch them out occasionally.

This box will get hot, so do not use this on a wooden deck or near anything flammable. Do not use this oven indoors as you will risk carbon monoxide poisoning.

Bonus Project: Spiral Hot Dogs

When grilling hot dogs, I feel that spiral cut hot dogs are something a little extra—they look neat, and they hold the hot dog condiments much better.

To spiral cut hot dogs, place the hot dog on a cutting board and hold a knife at a slight angle (the bigger the angle the wider the cut).

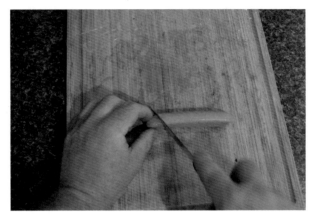

Figure 14.8 The bigger the angle the wider the cut.

Cut about 1/3 through the hot dog and roll it away from you while cutting—this will act like screwing a nut on a bolt and the knife will move along the hot dog. Do not cut all the way through the dog.

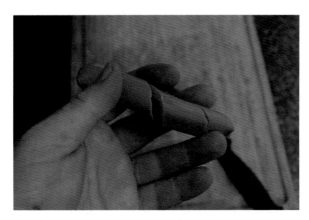

Figure 14.9 Don't cut all the way through.

As the hot dog cooks it will plump and the slices will open up.

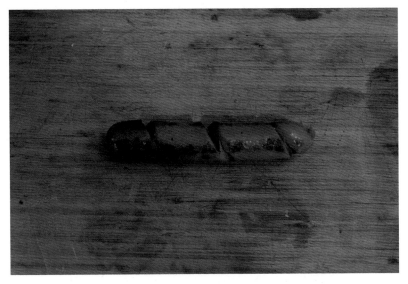

Figure 14.10 The slices will open during grilling.

Project 15: Cooking Bread in a Grill

One of the main reasons I write books like this is to help promote the notion that anyone can solve their problems with a little out of the box thinking. This is one example. Most people think that you require an oven to bake bread. Not true—all you need is a source of steady and controllable heat.

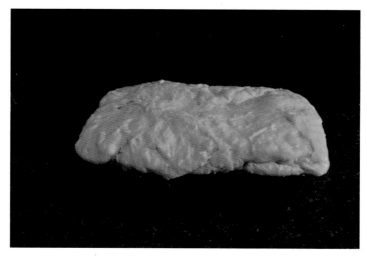

Figure 15.1 Bread can be baked anywhere you can get controlled heat.

Once you learn how to separate requirements from results, you will be surprised at how many ways you can get the job done.

The big thing to remember with baking on a grill is that it is hottest near the flames, so elevate the bread (even if you need to improvise).

Another important thing to note is that to bake perfect bread you need to be able to control both time and temperature. Since most grills have a thermometer on them, you should have it under control. If you don't, you may need to add a thermometer, or experiment until you learn just the right sized fire for your recipe.

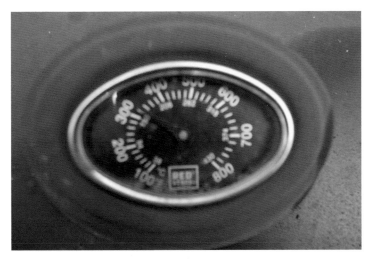

Figure 15.2 A grill thermometer is adequate for a good bread.

Rolls and buns will probably bake in 15–20 minutes and loaves will take 20–30 minutes, depending on their size and the grill's temperature.

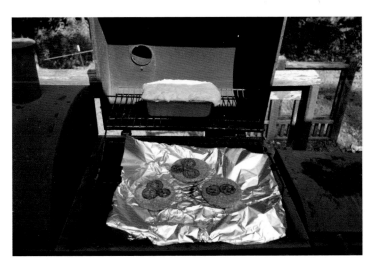

Figure 15.3 Depending on your grill, you may need to bake your bread on the top rack.

If you are making an entire meal, either to show off during a barbeque or in some grid down emergency, timing is important. Cook the bread before the meat.

This allows the bread to cool. Additionally, the grease from cooking meat makes the temperature unstable, and the smoke and soot from burning grease can stain your bread.

Grills don't circulate air as well as ovens do, which can lead to uneven heating. You may need to rotate your bread halfway through baking to have even cooking.

There is also a tendency for flames to burn the bottom of the bread, so keep the flames low and the bread elevated on a rack.

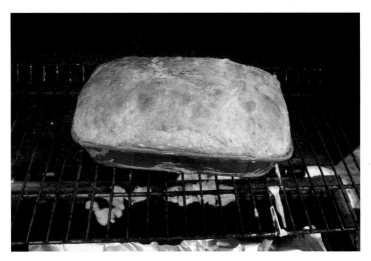

Figure 15.4 Grilled bread tastes wonderful.

Project 16: Canning Pickles

Many beginners who learn to can start with pickles. Pickles are a high acid food so it is safe to can them in a water bath. The recipe is also extremely simple, the materials inexpensive, and the end result is worth the effort.

Once the basics are mastered, almost anything can be pickled. As a matter of fact, when I was taking the pictures for this project, I went ahead and pickled some jalapeno peppers as well as some onions. I have a batch of pickled celery in my fridge waiting to be mixed with some tuna fish to make a delicious sandwich.

Pickling has been used for over 4,000 years and was one of the first safe methods of preserving out of season food.

The big things you need to know from a food safety standpoint are:

- Do not alter the proportions of vinegar/water/food.
- Do not use vinegar of unknown acidity—you need a pH of 4.6 or lower.
- You must have a minimum and uniform level of acidity throughout the food (which is why there are no guaranteed safe recipes for home pickling eggs since there is no way to ensure that the acid has gone to the center of the yolk).

Additionally, when using cucumbers, make sure you cut off at least $\frac{1}{16}$ of the blossom end of fresh cucumbers because the blossom end contains an enzyme that makes the pickles turn excessively soft.

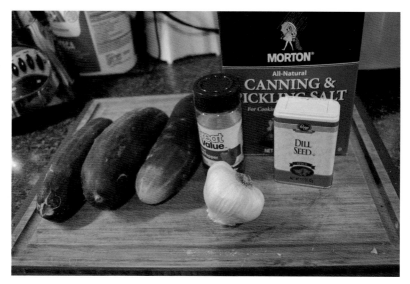

Figure 16.1 The ingredients

Ingredients:

- 8–10 small pickling cucumbers (about 3 pounds)
- 2 cups white vinegar
- 2 cups water
- 2 tablespoons pickling salt
- 4 heads fresh dill or 4 teaspoons dill seeds
- 4 small cloves garlic
- 1 tablespoon of red pepper flakes and/or black pepper (optional)

Equipment:

- 1 large pot (glass, enameled, or stainless steel—otherwise the acids may interact with the metal and produce an off taste)
- 1 water bath canner
- 4 pint canning jars with lids and sterile rings
- Large spoon and/or ladle
- Jar grabber
- Jar funnel

Procedure:

1. Combine vinegar, water, and salt in a saucepan and bring to a boil.
2. Place 1 sliced garlic clove, 1 teaspoon of dill seed (or a head of fresh dill) in the bottom of each jar. If you wish to use pepper flakes or black pepper, place ¼ tablespoon in the jars as well.

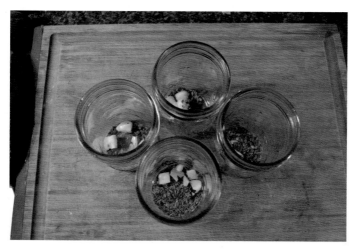

Figure 16.2 Place garlic and spices at bottom of jar.

3. Cut off blossom end of cucumber and slice them into spears.
4. Pack cucumber spears into the jars.

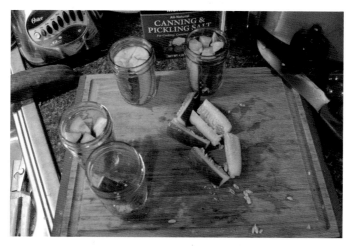

Figure 16.3 Cut into spears and place in jars.

5. Pour boiling vinegar mix over cucumbers and fill until ½ an inch from the top of the jar.
6. Tighten rings over jar lids and place filled jars in the water bath canner and ensure the canner is filled at least 1 inch over the tops of the jars. Use warm water to fill, as cold water may crack the jars since they will be warm from the boiling pickling solution.
7. Process the jars by boiling. If you use pint jars boil for 10 full minutes, and 15 if you are substituting pint jars with quart jars.

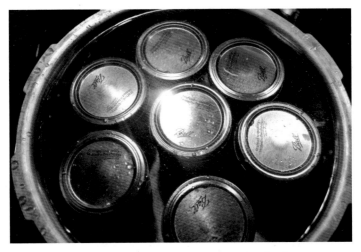

Figure 16.4 Process in boiling water bath.

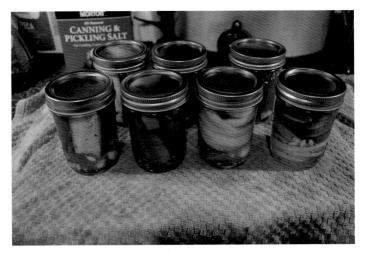

Figure 16.5 Finished pickles

Yield:
  4 pint jars of pickles

Notes:

- Processing longer than required will result in soggy pickles.
- The garlic may take on a blue or green tint due to the effect of the acid.
- Use pickling salt as the additives in table salt can discolor homemade pickles.
- You must use the correct amount of acid even though this will result in a sour pickle. You may add up to one tablespoon of sugar to use sweetness to counteract the sour taste.

Project 17:
Essene Bread

This is a very healthy, easy, and inexpensive food item. This is a primitive sprouted grain bread that raw food proponents eat uncooked or slightly heated. It gets its name from a second-century Jewish religious group called the Essenes and the recipe can be found in a first-century Aramaic manuscript called the Essene Gospel of Peace.

Because this is cooked very lightly and the only ingredients are water and sprouted grain, it is highly nutritious and can fit into almost any diet.

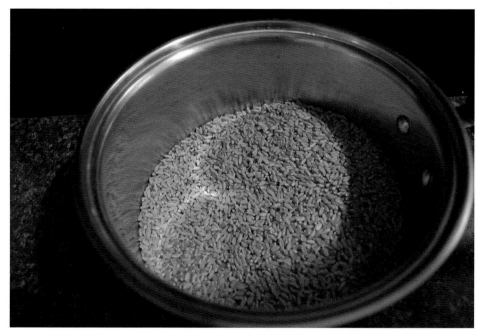

Figure 17.1 The main ingredient is wheat berries.

Ingredients:

- 2–4 cups wheat sprouts (sprout root should be approximately equal in length to the wheat berry)

Equipment:

- Sprouter (I use a deep bowl to sprout this much wheat at a time.)
- Wheat grinder
- Cookie sheet

Preparation:

1. Sprout the wheat by soaking overnight in chlorine free water, draining, and keeping damp for several days until the sprouts are the appropriate length. I get good results when I cover it with water and drain twice a day for about 4 days.

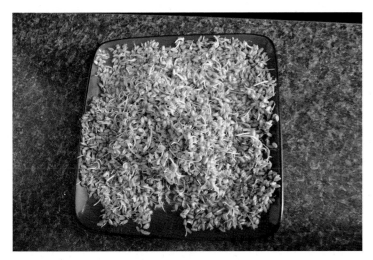

Figure 17.2 Sprouted wheat

2. Grind the sprouts. The wheat should be damp but not wet. I normally skip the last soak/drain step before I actually grind the sprouts. Damp sprouts will actually come out of the grinder as a wet paste.

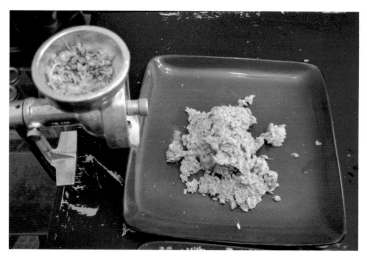

Figure 17.3 Grind the sprouts.

3. Wet your hands and form the dough into oval or round loaves, balls, sticks, or buns. Use parchment paper, or coat the bottom of the loaf in sesame seeds, oats, or wheat berries or it *will* stick to the pan.

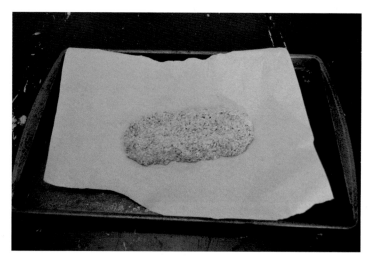

Figure 17.4 Shape into loaf.

4. Always use a cookie sheet and bake at approximately 160°F. Time depends on the size of the loaf. The loaf pictured turned a nice brown after about 30 minutes. The idea is to have a nice brown crispy outside but to keep a moist center.

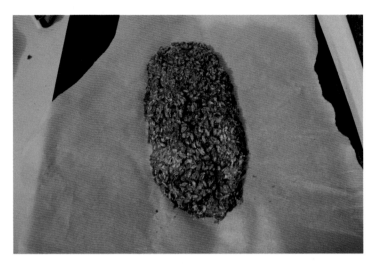

Figure 17.5 Tastes like a whole wheat cracker on the outside crust, and fresh whole wheat on the inside.

Yield:

One small loaf, which will feed 2 adults for a single meal

Notes:

The sprouting process causes an increase in vitamins, minerals, and other essential nutrients.

You do not need to knead the dough, although a little kneading produces a better loaf.

The bread will not rise, so you can go straight from grinding and molding to the oven.

Project 18:
Box Fan Dehydrator

I was looking for a way to make a homemade dehydrator and lucked into this one made from a box fan—I like it because, unlike all my other dehydrators, it does not take up a lot of room in my yard (solar) or on my shelf (all the others). It doesn't take up room because when I am not using it as a dehydrator, it pulls double duty as a box fan.

After I saw this on several prepper/food blogs, I realized that it was also on an episode of *Good Eats* with Alton Brown. I miss that show, as they always had good ideas (like this one apparently).

No matter where it came from, this is a cool way to start learning to dehydrate as it does not take any special tools and you can improvise and try new ways of doing things. Personally, I think the air filter part is begging for some modification—maybe some window screen or a box with a tulle cover?

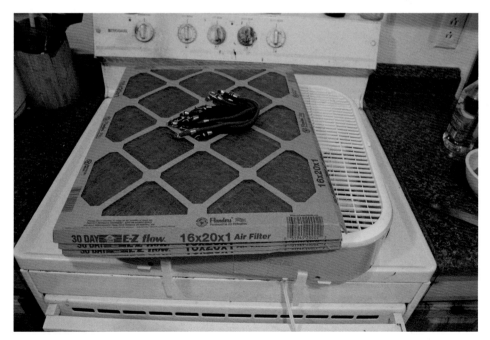

Figure 18.1 The materials

Materials:

- One 20 inch x 20 inch box fan
- 4 cotton-based air filters (cotton fiber is best; do not use hepa filters)
- 2 bungee cords
- Whatever you wish to dehydrate

Procedure:

1. Prepare your food items—if wet, blot dry; if thick, slice thin, and season as appropriate.
2. Lay food in a single layer on 3 of the 4 air filters. Ensure they do not touch.

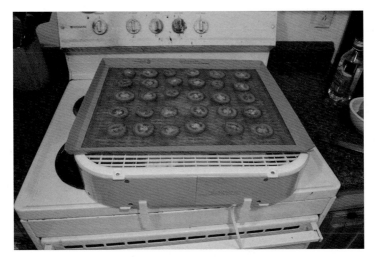

Figure 18.2 Stack food on filters.

3. Stack food-layered filters on top of each other, no more than three filters high.
4. Use the fourth filter to cover the food so it does not fall off when you attach the filters to the fan.
5. Turn the fan so that it is lying motor side down with the direction of the airflow facing upwards.

6. Set the filter/food sandwich on the fan, with the channels in the filter orientated side to side so that when you stand the filter up, the channels run parallel to the floor. (This keeps the food from sliding down.)

7. Attach the two bungee cords to the side of the fan, pull them across the filters, and attach to the other side of the fan.

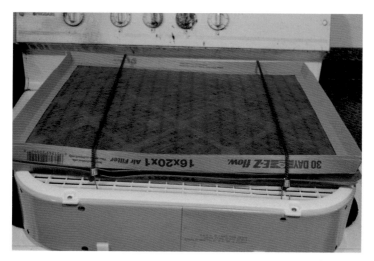

Figure 18.3 Bungee cords tie filters to fan.

8. Take the fan someplace where dogs or other animals will not rip through the paper to get to your food.

9. Stand the fan up and turn on.

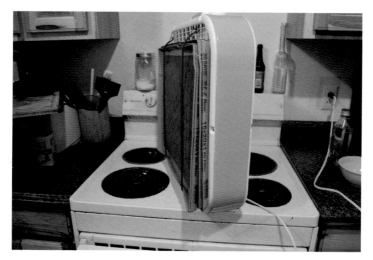

Figure 18.4 Turn up and turn on.

10. Items like beef jerky should take 12–14 hours, but begin to check your food every hour after about 6 hours.

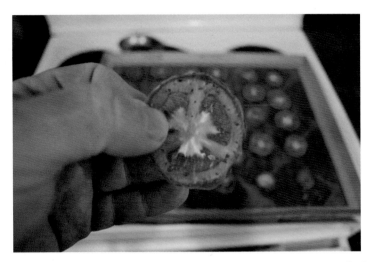

Figure 18.5 Run until the food reaches the moisture content you desire.

Yield:
Varies

Project 19:

Dehydrated Tomatoes Packed in Oil (Sun-Dried Tomato Clone)

Dehydrated tomatoes packed in oil are a great way to extend your tomato season. Besides being a great food preservation item, they taste really good in salads and pasta dishes. The best thing about this recipe is that dehydrating enhances the tomato flavor, which makes the soft oil-soaked tomatoes great for adding flavor to food storage.

This is a very simple recipe that is easier than actually growing the tomatoes.

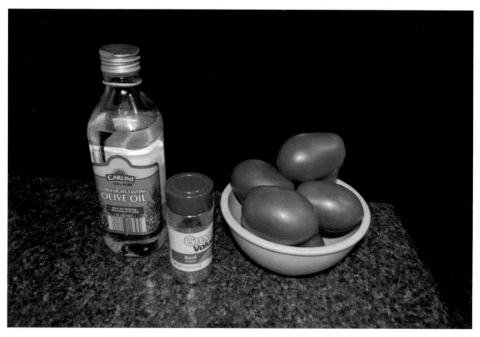

Figure 19.1 The ingredients

Ingredients:

- Tomatoes (Yield varies depending upon the moisture inside the tomatoes. Paste tomatoes like Roma are best and typically yield 2 cups of dried tomatoes for each 5 pounds of fresh fruit.)
- Olive oil
- Spices (garlic, basil, salt)

Equipment:

One of the following:

- Oven *or*
- Food dehydrator *or*
- Car on a hot sunny day

Procedure:

1. Slice the tomatoes.

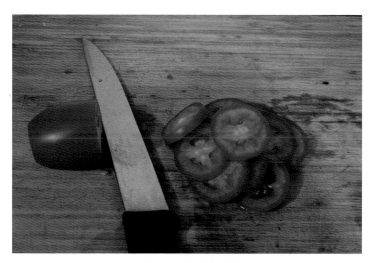

Figure 19.2 Slice thin.

2. Season the tomatoes with sea salt, kosher salt, and/or some spices (typically basil) if desired.

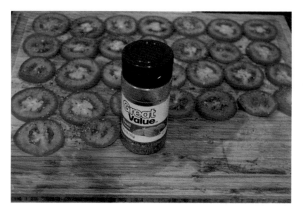

Figure 19.3 Season as desired.

3. Dry until leathery but not until crispy. The first time I tried this recipe I dehydrated the tomatoes until they would snap apart and they never achieved the soft texture of good oil-packed sun-dried tomato.

   a. Food dehydrator: Arrange the pieces on each rack so that air can circulate. If your food drier has a thermostat, set it for 140°F. It will take 3 to 8 hours.

   b. Oven: Preheat the oven to 150°F (or warm). Arrange the tomatoes on cake racks. Cookie sheets will work if you don't have cake racks or screens, but you need to flip or stir the tomatoes once in a while to expose the other side of them. Close the oven. It takes about 10–20 hours and you will need to check them often. You may need to rotate the shelves and move them up or down to get even heating.

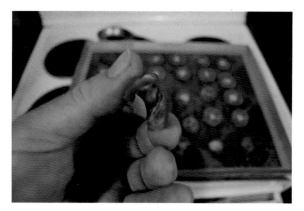

Figure 19.4 Dry until flexible, not until brittle.

    c. Automobile and a hot day: Spread the tomato slices out on shallow trays. Put the trays on the dashboard of your car and roll all the windows up and park in the sunniest spot you've got. It may take a couple of days to dry, if so bring the tomatoes in the house overnight.

4. Fill a mason jar with the slices and top with oil until 1 inch from the top of the jar. (I also like to throw in a little basil and garlic in the jar.)

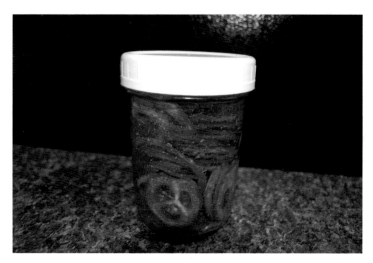

Figure 19.5 Pack in oil.

Project 20:
Biltong (South African Cured Meat Jerky)

Biltong is cured meat from South Africa. Like jerky, it is both a technique and a description of a food product. Also like jerky, Biltong can be made with many different types of meat, from beef to ostrich.

Generally, Biltong is made from raw fillets of meat that are cut into strips just like jerky. However, Biltong is much thicker (one inch in some cases—which is much thicker than the typical ⅛-inch-thick jerky strips). The spice mix used to create Biltong is also different, as it normally contains vinegar.

Biltong was developed to preserve meat in the hostile South African environment without the need for refrigeration.

Besides the unique taste, Biltong is a good method for food preservation as it is very easy to prepare—but first you need to make a Biltong box to dry the meat. Luckily, it is quite easy to do.

The goal of a Biltong box is to provide a place to dry your meat, while allowing air flow and preventing flies from getting to your meat.

We are going to make a simple biltong box using a plastic bin. The process is simple enough for you to easily reconfigure the instructions to make a cheaper cardboard box or a more durable wooden box.

Biltong Box

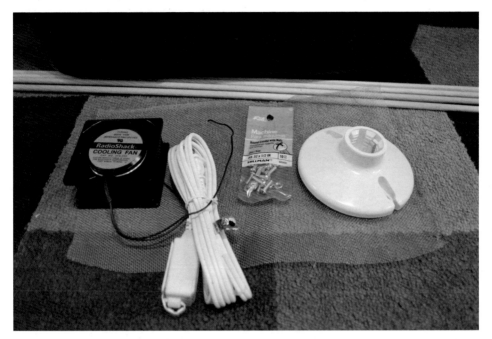

Figure 20.1 The materials

Materials:

- 1 sealable plastic container (deep enough to hang meat and tight enough to keep out flies)
- 9 lengths of dowel rod (I was able to cut 3 long dowels into 3 equal sections each for 9 rods.)
- 1 small fan
- Screen for fan
- 1 light fitting
- 1 40-watt light bulb (incandescent—you need the heat)
- Wire
- 3-prong plug
- Machine nuts and screws

Procedure:

1. Put the top on the container to ensure that the holes you are going to drill for the dowels do not interfere with a tight closing lid.

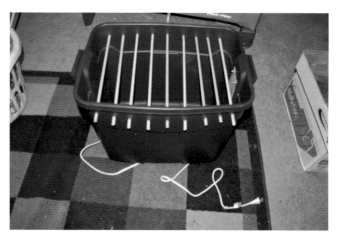

Figure 20.2 Dowels should not interfere with lid closing.

2. Mark and drill holes on both sides of the container (longways) so that the 7 dowels are parallel and equally spaced down the long side of the container.
3. On the narrow end of the container, drill a hole near a corner near the bottom of the box to fit the cord for the light that will be inside the box.

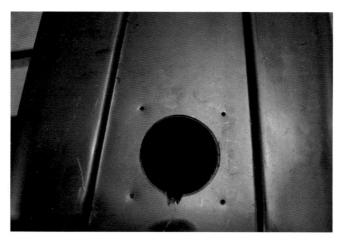

Figure 20.3 Drill hole for fan.

4. Next to the light, in the other corner, drill a hole and mount the fan on the outside of box, oriented to blow air into the box.

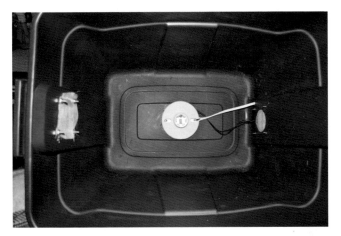

Figure 20.4 Mount the light and fan.

5. On the other narrow end of the box, opposite the light and fan but near the top of the box, drill a hole to allow air to escape.

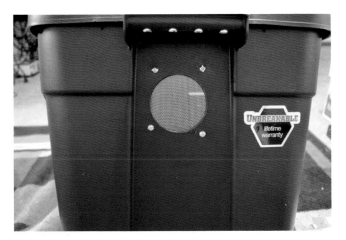

Figure 20.5 Screened vent hole, diagonally situated from inlet fan

6. Affix screen to the fan and the outlet holes to keep flies and other vermin out of the box.
7. Thoroughly clean the inside of the box and ensure it is completely dry before hanging meat in the box.

Biltong Recipe

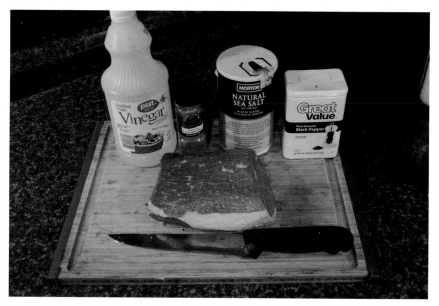

Figure 20.6 The ingredients

Ingredients:

- 4 pounds chunk of eye round
- 2 tablespoons of ground black pepper
- ½ cup coarsely ground roasted coriander
- 2 tablespoons sea salt
- 1 cup vinegar

Equipment:

- Wide tray
- Sharp knife
- Measuring cup
- Clean towel
- Paperclips

Procedure:

1. Mix the spices and vinegar together.
2. Pour a portion of the vinegar spice mix in the bottom of the tray to create a thin layer of vinegar.

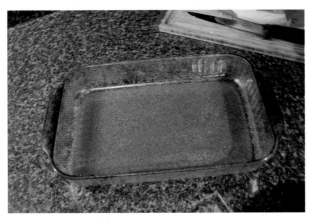

Figure 20.7 Cover bottom of tray with vinegar spice mix.

3. Cut meat along the grain, into inch-and-a-bit thick slices.
4. Put meat slices into tray.
5. Cover meat with the vinegar mix, cover with box lid, and let sit overnight.
6. Unbend paperclips to form a "S" shaped hook.
7. Skewer one end of each meat slice with a paperclip, and hang over dowel rods.

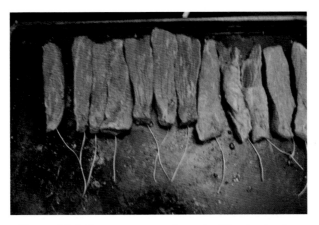

Figure 20.8 Skewer seasoned meat with wire hooks.

8. Hang until dried to taste. The dryer the meat, the better it will store, but Biltong is traditionally left "wetter" than jerky—this can take from 1–10 days depending on taste, ambient temperature, and humidity.

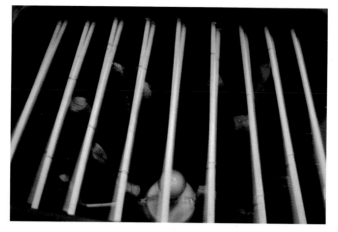

Figure 20.9 Hang until dried.

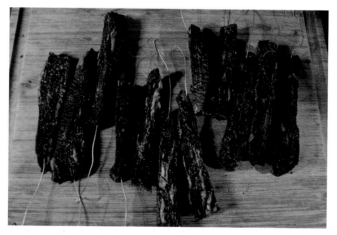

Figure 20.10 Biltong is traditionally not dried as much as jerky, so it is much thicker.

Yield:
Approximately 16 servings

Project 21: Potting Meat

This project is a "if everything else fails" method. Potting meat is an ancient food storage technique that worked for thousands of years; however, the USDA recommends against this process because of the potential for botulism.

Personally, I would rather pressure can meat since it is much safer. However, crocking meat is still used as a culinary practice in France.

Potting (also known as crocking) meat is a process where meat is fully cooked, placed in a sterile ceramic container, and then covered with melted fat. When the fat solidifies, the crock is covered and stored in a cool and dry location.

The idea is that the cooking destroys any bacteria in the meat and the fat covering seals the meat so that no new contamination can occur. This is a similar process to canning in that the fat seals the meat from recontamination of bacteria, just like the can and lid does.

Like canning, care must be taken to properly cook the meat because the fat can insulate botulism spores that were not destroyed—thereby locking them in the perfect conditions to grow (just like canning jars).

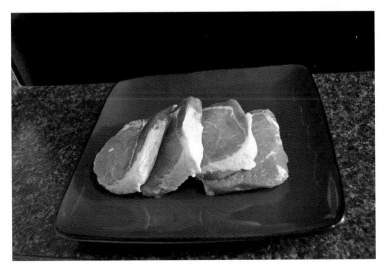

Figure 21.1 The ingredients

Ingredients:

- Meat (I used pork chops, which are perfect for crocking, but sausage or bacon also work well.)
- Fat (amount depends on the size of the crock and the amount of the meat, but I used a medium-sized container of Manteca (pork fat).

Equipment:

- Skillet
- Pot
- Ceramic crock
- Tongs

Procedure:

1. Thoroughly clean a ceramic crock with very hot soapy water. Items cannot be sterile until they are clean.
2. Sterilize by pouring boiling water into the crock. Hold the hot water in the crock until just before filling with meat.

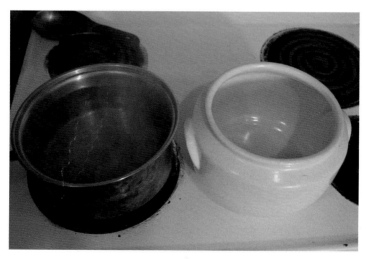

Figure 21.2 Boiling water to sterilize crock.

3. While water is boiling, melt some fat in a clean pot so you have enough grease to cover all the meat completely.

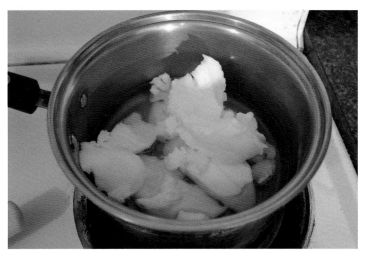

Figure 21.3 Melt lard.

4. Completely cook meat until the internal temperature is above 250ºF.

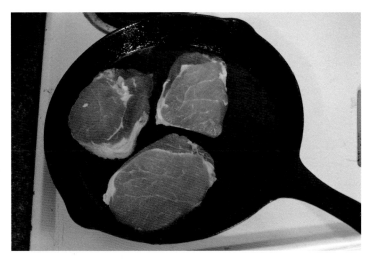

Figure 21.4 Cook until completely done.

5. Empty the water from the crock and wipe the crock dry with a clean towel.

6. Place hot grease in the bottom of the crock so that the bottom of the crock is covered.
7. Place a layer of cooked meat into the crock.

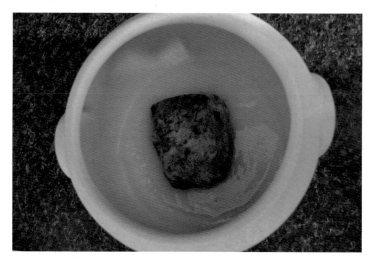

Figure 21.5 Layer meat on top of grease.

8. Cover with hot grease.
9. Add another layer of meat and repeat adding hot grease.
10. When the crock is full or you run out of meat, cover the meat with at least 2–3 inches of hot grease.

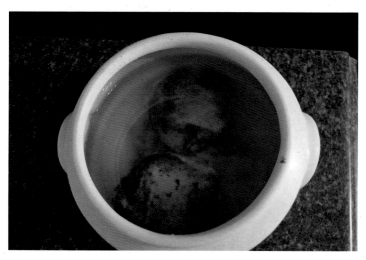

Figure 21.6 Full crock

11. Cover the crock with a plate or a cloth. Store the crock in a cool, dry place.

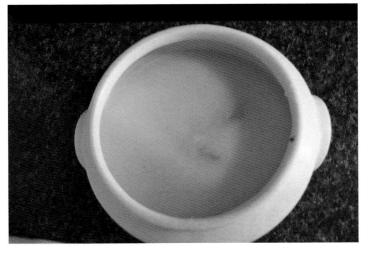

Figure 21.7 Hardened fat is fully covering meat.

12. When you want to eat your pork chops, remove the meat carefully. Place in a frying pan and re-fry and heat thoroughly. You want the internal temperature of the meat to reach at least 250ºF again.

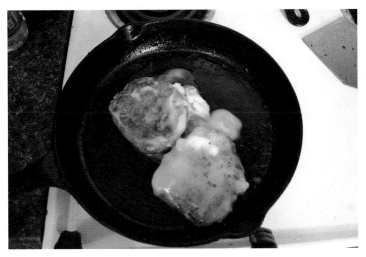

Figure 21.8 Reheat crocked meat.

Yield:

Variable

Note:

I believe that crocked meat is superior in flavor and taste to canned sausage patties or links. However, as with all things stored, you must trust your nose and other senses when cooking stored food. If anything seems off, discard the food.

Project 22: Cultivator Disk Grill "Disco"

My first encounter with a Disco was a few months ago when I was reading a fiction book. The hero was hiding from rogue military operatives on a ranch and was fed using something called a "discada"—a couple minutes of Internet research introduced me into the wild world of the Cowboy Wok, Disco, or Discada.

Basically, a disco is a concave griddle made of an old cultivator plow disk with the center hole welded shut, some handles welded on, and the whole thing cleaned up and seasoned like you would a cast iron skillet.

There are all sorts of recipes that use a disco and the term discada is used in the southwest like BBQ is used in my home state of Tennessee, both as a noun and a verb.

After building and using a disco, I am sure that the reason the cowboy wok is not used universally is that the shipping cost and availability of the cultivator disks are prohibitively expensive in areas that do not have the appropriate agriculture infrastructure.

I really wanted a 3-foot disk to use over a campfire, but shipping costs were enormous. I had to settle with a 28-inch disk I bought at my local farmer's co-op.

Making a discada is pretty simple; if you live in Texas you can purchase a disk that has not had the center mounting hole punched in. Otherwise, you need to cut a piece of steel to fit the hole and weld it in place. I used a bit of an old lawnmower blade.

I would imagine that if you lacked the ability to weld, and did not want to pay a machine shop to weld in a plug, you could use a hiller disk, which has four small mounting bolts, but it is not as big or as deep. If you were careful, you could even use a disco with a center hole, but you would lose a lot of fat to the fire.

I decided to weld handles to the side of my grill. I used horseshoes as is typically done by most Texans, but anything can work as long as it is sturdy.

Next, I used a drill with a wire wheel to remove any rust, coatings, and grease that were on my disk.

After wiping the disk down with an alcohol-soaked rag, I washed it with soapy water, let dry, and then seasoned it with lard just as you would a cast iron skillet.

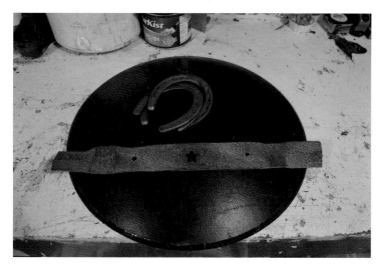

Figure 22.1 The materials

Materials:

- Cultivator disk (If you do not have a welder you can use a Hiller disk which has 4 small bolt holes instead of the large center mounting hole—but they are not as large or as deep.)
- 2 horseshoes
- 2 x 2 block of metal to plug hole (I used a bit of a lawnmower blade.)
- Oil and charcoal for seasoning

Equipment:

- Cutting wheel or hacksaw
- Sandpaper
- Grinder
- Welder (or $20 to pay a welding shop to plug the hole)

Procedure:

1. Cut a plug to fit in the center hole of the cultivator disk.

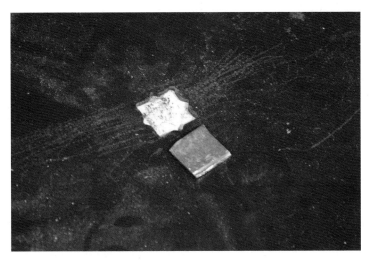

Figure 22.2 Hole and metal plug

2. Remove the painted coating to ensure both a good weld and a safe food surface.

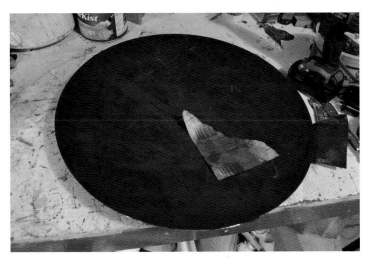

Figure 22.3 It took a *lot* of sandpaper, and my hands were coated in black crud.

3. Weld the plug into place. If you cannot weld, a local mechanic would probably do it for you for around $20, some beer, or an invite to the first cookout.
4. Weld the handles in place. I used two for simplicity, but I plan on making another with three so that I can hang it over the fire on a tripod.
5. Grind the weld marks down to ensure a flat surface. You don't want to grind any more than you need, as the machine marking on the inside of the disk helps hold food in place and is essential to stir frying.

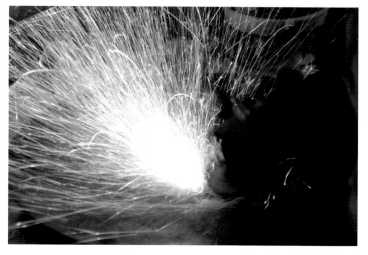

Figure 22.4 Go easy on the grinder.

6. Burn off any residue before you season just like you would to restore an old cast iron skillet. I filled the disk with charcoal, ignited it, let it burn itself to ash, and then let the disco cool slowly.
7. Season the disco before use, then handle just as you would a cast iron skillet.

To Season:

1. Heat disco to a high temperature, around 300°F.

2. Coat with lard, corn oil, or bacon fat.

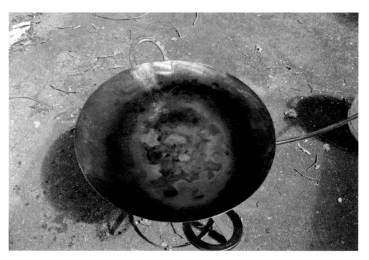

Figure 22.5 Heat evenly and coat with oil.

3. Rub melted fat onto all areas of the grill.
4. Let cool.
5. Repeat as needed.

Beef Discada

Ingredients:
- 2 chopped onions
- 5 sliced peppers
- 2 cloves minced garlic
- 1.5 pounds beef round
- oil

Equipment:
- Disco
- Turkey fryer, round grill, or hole with large rocks
- Spatula
- Oil
- Salt
- Rag

Procedure:
1. Heat disco with oil until a drop of water sizzles when dropped onto the center of grill.
2. Place onions in center of disco and cook until they start to soften and caramelize.
3. Dump your peppers and garlic into the grill and mix with onions. Cook peppers until the peppers start to turn soft.
4. Lastly throw the meat into the center of the grill and cook until done to your preference.
5. Once the mix is cooked and removed from grill, let the disco cool and clean with oil and salt. Once seasoned, never let soap touch the grill or the seasoning will be removed. Never store dirty, or without a light coating of vegetable or other food grade oil.

Yield:

4–5 Adults

Notes:

The Internet abounds with disco recipes. There is one recipe that claims to feed 78 people for $10; but it basically consists of throwing hot dogs, spam, and every other cheap meat in with the beef and peppers as a means to stretch the expensive ingredients.

This method of cooking is very flexible and is more about getting out and having fun, rather than following a specific set of instructions.

You may find that it is easier to locate a repair shop to weld the disk rather than to do it yourself. I was able to get mine to stick, but I ended up using the experience of a friend of mine to finish it out.

Project 23: Biosand Filter

This project is a technique that has been used to treat water for more than two hundred years. While using sand and gravel to filter water seems simple, this system uses multiple mechanisms to kill, trap, or remove bacteria.

A biosand filter is simple to operate, cheap, easy to build, and it can be quite effective. Its biggest drawbacks are its stationary nature, the continuous nature of filtering, and the fact that it takes a few weeks to begin to operate at peak efficiency. This type of filter works extremely well for removing sediment, algae, and biological pathogens, but it does not work well to remove chemical pollutants.

A biosand filter (BSF) is basically layered sand and gravel in a watertight container. The top layer of sand removes pathogens and suspended solids from drinking water. The gravel allows the water to settle at the bottom of the container and to be drawn out through a perforated pipe. Additionally, over time, a community of bacteria called the biolayer grows in the top inch of sand. This biolayer eats much of the bad bacteria that live in polluted water.

Pathogens and suspended solids are removed through biological and physical processes that take place in the sand. These processes include mechanical trapping, predation, adsorption, and natural death.

The biosand filter has been studied in the field for decades, and has been shown in laboratory testing to remove:

- Up to 100 percent of helminths (worms)
- Up to 100 percent of protozoa
- Up to 98.5 percent of bacteria
- 70–99 percent of viruses

The filter can also remove up to 95 percent of turbidity (dirt and cloudiness) and up to 95 percent of iron.

A simple biofilter can be made using some plumbing fittings, 2 five-gallon food grade buckets, a bag of fine sand, and a small amount of gravel. Once you understand the process, you can scale this filter up or down to fit your needs.

Additionally, some filters are built with a layer of charcoal between the sand and gravel to further remove contaminants from the water, but this is not strictly necessary.

Materials:

- 2 food grade buckets with tight-fitting lids
- Fine sand
- Gravel
- 3 ft PVC pipe (½-inch or ¾-inch—the size of the pipe does not matter as much, as long as it fits the valve you will use)
- Valve with o-ring and bulkhead nut
- PVC Fittings

    ○ One "T"
    ○ 2 90-degree elbows
    ○ 2 caps

- PVC cement
- 4 stainless steel ¼-inch bolts 1 inch long with 2 washers and one nut each

Tools:

- Small nail or ⅛-inch or smaller drill bit
- Drill
- ¼-inch drill bit
- Spade bit appropriate for a tight fit of your valve
- Adjustable wrench
- Saw
- Dremel tool with cutting blade is optional*

Procedure:

1. Flip one bucket upside down and center one bucket lid (also upside down) on it.
2. Drill 4 ¼-inch holes approximately one inch from edge of the bucket (not the lid) through both the lid and the bottom of the bucket.

They should be orientated as corners of a square; or, if you were looking at a map, North, South, East, and West.

3. Bolt the lid to the bottom of the bucket using the 4 bolts and washers. Depending on the buckets you may need to run a bead of silicon sealant around the bottom of the bucket so that water does not leak over the top of the lid.

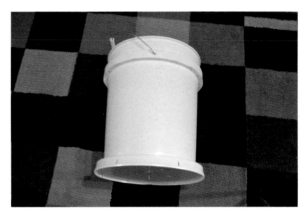

Figure 23.1 Attach lid to bottom of bucket.

4. Drill multiple ⅛-inch holes through the lid and bucket assembly, taking care not to drill holes in the lid only. This forms a diffuser so that water can drip into the filter slowly and without disturbing the biolayer. Alternatively, you can heat the small nail with a torch and use pliers to poke 30–40 holes in the plastic buckets; but I find that drilling is faster and easier.

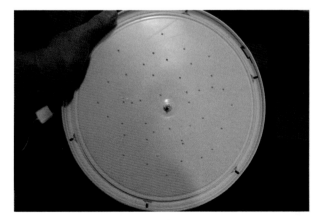

Figure 23.2 Drill many small holes through bottom of bucket and the attached lid.

5. Set this assembly aside.
6. Using the second bucket, measure your valve to see how far up the valve needs to be on the side of the bucket to clear the bucket base. The lower you can install the valve, the better.
7. Drill a hole in the side of the second bucket and push the valve through the hole.
8. Cut a 2- to 3-inch piece of pipe to fit on the valve inside the bucket, and insert the short piece of pipe into the opening in the center of the PCV "T."*

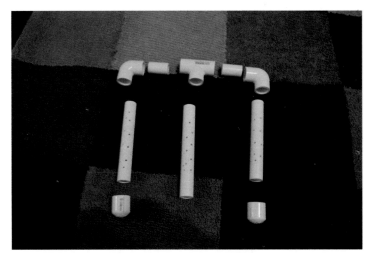

Figure 23.3 PVC fittings setup

9. Cut two 3- to 4-inch pieces of pipe and insert one in the ends of the PVC "T."
10. Insert an elbow on the ends of the 2 3- to 4-inch pipe sections.
11. Cut the remaining length of pipe in half, and insert each into the open end of the elbows—the PVC assembly should look like a block "E."

12. Screw the valve into the side of the bucket, and insert the center of the "E" into the valve. Ensure that the pipe assembly fits easily in the bottom of the bucket.*

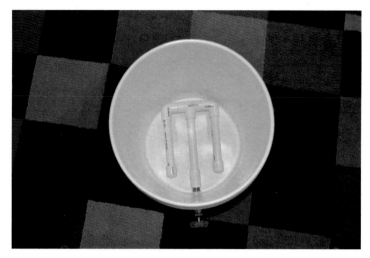

Figure 23.4 Test fit and remove.

13. Remove assembly and drill multiple ⅛-inch holes in the pipes randomly around the circumference of the pipe. You could also use a dremel tool to cut thin slots in the pipe (which works better in my experience, but is easier to mess up). These openings allow water to flow out of the filter with the valve open.

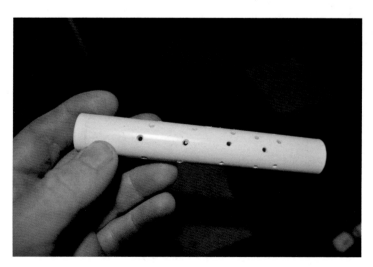

Figure 23.5 Drill small holes in the filter assembly pipes.

14. If everything fits, glue the pipes together, and then glue the pipe assembly to the valve.
15. Cover the pipe assembly with loose gravel—about ½–1 inch above the pipe is fine.

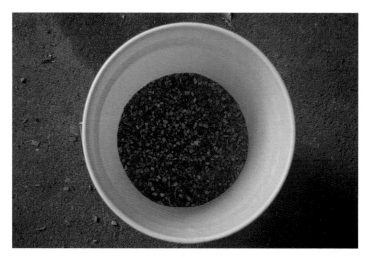

Figure 23.6 Cover with loose gravel (I use live pea gravel, as limestone gravel can add dissolved minerals to the water).

16. Fill bucket to about 5–6 inches from the top of the bucket with clean fine sand.

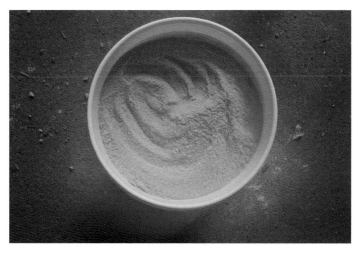

Figure 23.7 Top gravel with clean sand.

17. Close valve and fill with water.
18. Cover water-filled bucket with the lid/bucket assembly from step 1, and ensure lid is tightly snapped on bottom bucket.
19. Fill top bucket with water.

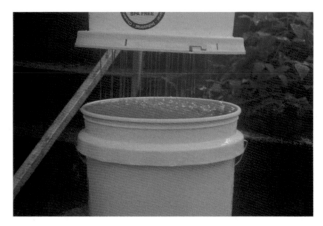

Figure 23.8 You want the water to flow gently through many holes—like rain.

20. It is vital that the sand is always kept covered by at least an inch of water. If the top layer of sand dries out, the beneficial bacterium that eats the pathogenic bacteria will die.
21. Set the filter buckets on a stand, open the valve, and let the water slowly drip into a collection bucket.

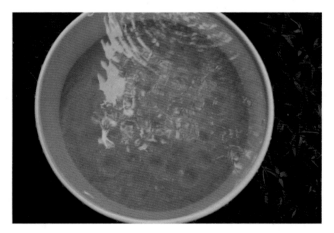

Figure 23.9 The water flow should be gentle enough not to wash away or destroy the bacteria film that will develop over time.

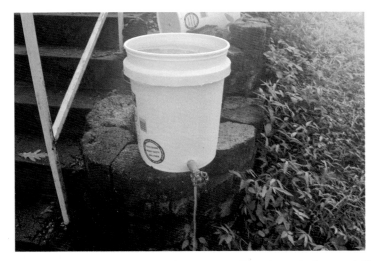

Figure 23.10 It will not take long for water to flow through the sand filter.

22. When the collection bucket gets close to full, dump the water back into the top bucket. After a few days of recycling the water, a biofilm of bacteria should have grown on the sand, and you can begin to use the filter.

*Do not glue the PVC fittings yet. Wait until you are sure the measurements work in your buckets.

This filter is best used as part of a larger water purification system, and boiling or chlorinating the filtered water should also be considered.

To use a biosand filter:

Contaminated water is poured into the top of the biosand filter at least once per day (taking care to diffuse the water, as a stream may erode a channel into the sand and destroy the effectiveness of the biolayer).

Treated water flows out of the outlet tube. No power is required—the filter works by gravity.

It should take about one hour to get 3–5 gallons of filtered drinking water.

Project 24:
Sterilizing Water in a Pressure Cooker

This method is much like pressure canning. Except instead of sterilizing food, we will be sterilizing drinking water in glass canning jars. Unlike filtering or distillation, this will not do anything for contaminants—just organisms.

To truly sterilize something, it must be *clean* and free of all microbes and spores.

Boiling does *not* kill all bacteria. Some bacteria are actually resistant to the temperature of boiling water at 212°F (100°C). Many bacteria form spores that can withstand boiling. To kill all the bacteria, you need to raise the temperature to about 250°F (121°C). Sterilizing with steam heat is the most common method to obtain this level of sterility. It is also the most effective, since spores can resist dry heat, but 30 minutes of exposure to steam at 250°F (121°C) will kill almost anything.

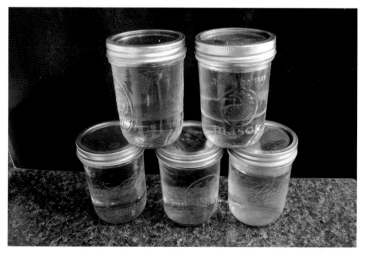

Figure 24.1 The finished product

Materials:

- Water
- Mason jars, lids, rings

Equipment:

- Pressure cooker
- Tongs
- Towel

Procedure:

1. Fill the canning jars with water, leaving 1 inch head space from the top before closing the lid, and only tightening the bands just finger tight.
2. Add approximately 2 inches of water to the pot.
3. Place the supporting rack inside.
4. Add the water-filled jars to the pot.

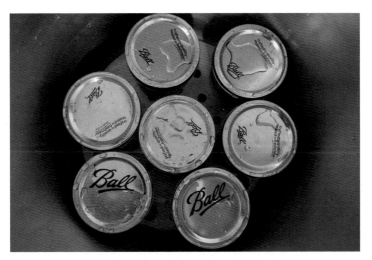

Figure 24.2 Fill canner with jars.

5. Lock the canner lid in place, but do *not* place the weight on the vent pipe.
6. Turn the heat to high.

7. As soon as the water at the bottom of the pot begins boiling the steam will displace the air inside the unit.
8. Let the steam escape from the cooker or canner in order to expel the air.
9. Wait until a good jet of steam is venting from the vent pipe before replacing the pressure regulator weight on the vent pipe.

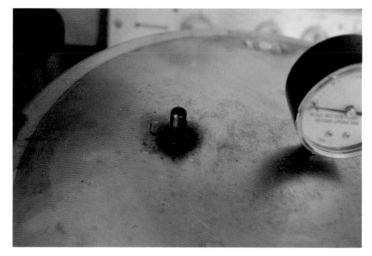

Figure 24.3 Wait until steam is blowing out of vent before placing weight.

10. Once the pressure setting reaches 15 psi, turn down the heat and start a 30 minute timer.

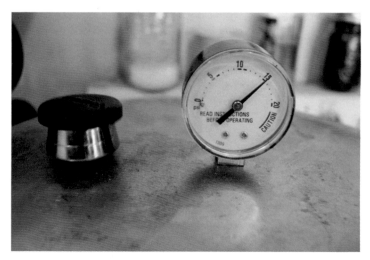

Figure 24.4 Process at 15 psi.

11. Make sure the pressure setting remains constant. If pressure drops, get back up to 15 psi and restart timer.
12. After 30 minutes, turn off the heat and allow the pot to cool naturally until the pressure slowly drops.
13. The jars of sterile water should now be removed immediately.

Note:

As long as the sterilized liquid remains sealed, the jars should be free of microbes until it is opened again.

It occurs to me that if you are having to sterilize water in a pressure cooker, the chances are that your kitchen stove isn't working. As a result, I have included instructions below on how to use a pressure cooker on a wood fire.

If your pressure cooker is stainless steel and does not have any sort of applied coating or nonstick finish, it can be heated outside over a wood or charcoal fire.

• Start by digging a shallow depression in the dirt and build a fire in it.
• Build up a large enough fire to produce a deep bed of coals.
• Position the canner in the heart of the coals.
• Move it in or out of the hottest part of the coals as needed.

Cooking on a fire is harder than on a stove because it will be necessary to reposition it in order to maintain proper pressure.

Project 25:

Caramel "Dulce de Leche"

This is something I have been meaning to try for several months, but could not quite decide what to make to put it *on*. However, once I made it I realized that a spoon is the perfect thing to douse liberally with this golden condiment.

This is very easy, with several ways of making it. I am going to show you two ways—one is easier (crock pot) and the other is faster (pressure cooker).

Ingredients:

• Evaporated milk

Equipment:

• Water
  And either
  Pressure cooker and steamer basket
  Or a
  Crock pot

Procedure:

Crock Pot Method:

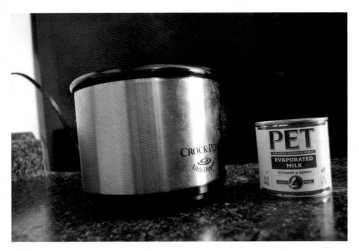

Figure 25.1 Crock Pot method

1. Fill crock pot with water.
2. Drop in unopened can of evaporated milk.

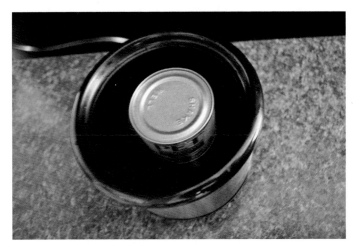

Figure 25.2 Cook on high for 8 hours.

3. Heat on high for 8 hours.
4. Let cool before opening the can.

Pressure Canner Method:

1. Fill pressure canner 2 inches deep with water.
2. Place steamer basket in bottom of canner (or any heat resistance object for the milk can to sit on without allowing it to touch the sides or bottom of canner).

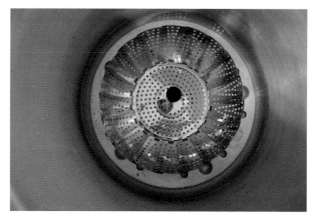

Figure 25.3 Put basket in canner.

3. Put unopened can in the basket (if the can touches the sides of the canner it may explode).

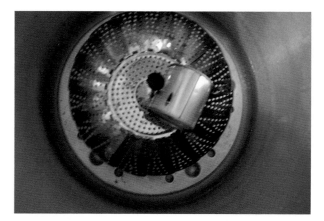

Figure 25.4 Keep can from sides or it may explode.

4. Close canner and process at 15 pounds for 15 minutes.
5. Let cool naturally and do not open can of milk until it is cool.

Yield:

One can of caramel

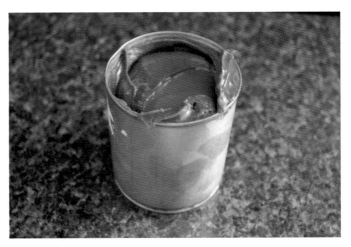

Figure 25.5 Sweet goodness

Note:

This is a great dessert ingredient that can be added to pies, ice cream, and all manner of goodness; but I like it with apples.

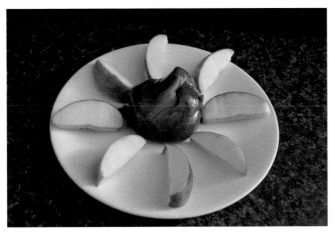

Figure 25.6 Great with apples

Project 26:
Making Ghee (Clarified Butter)

Ghee is clarified butter that has had a lot of the milk solids and lactose removed by heating. It can be stored in an airtight container without refrigeration for many months.

I like it because it has a very high smoke point (482°F), so it is perfect for frying.

It is also great on breads or anything else that you would typically spread butter on.

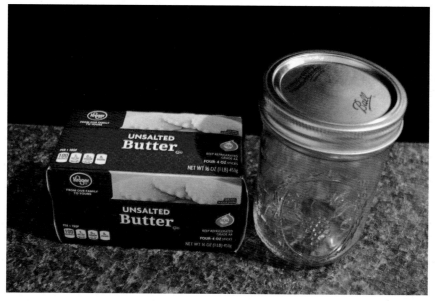

Figure 26.1 The ingredients

Ingredients:

- 1 lb unsalted butter (anything with a salty flavor will be intensified, so salted butter will be almost inedible)

Equipment:

- Saucepan
- Cheesecloth/rubber band
- Canning funnel
- Sterile pint mason jar/lid and ring

Procedure:

1. Melt the butter slowly on the stovetop over medium heat until it boils. It will foam.

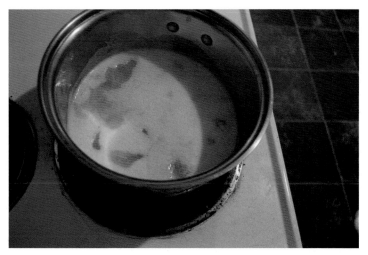

Figure 26.2 First foam

2. Once boiling, reduce heat to medium. The butter foam will subside.

3. As the butter clarifies, foam will form a second time. Ghee is done when the second foam forms large bubbles and the butter turns golden.

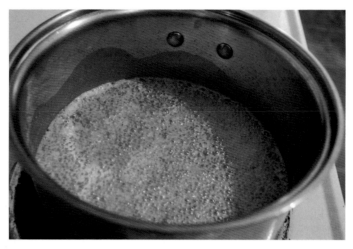

Figure 26.3 Large bubbles mean you are almost done.

4. You will need to strain the brown milk solids that are sitting in the bottom of pan.

   a. Insert a canning funnel into the mouth of a pint-sized sterile mason jar.
   b. Drape cheesecloth over the mouth of the funnel and hold in place with a rubber band.
   c. Gently pour the ghee through the cheesecloth.

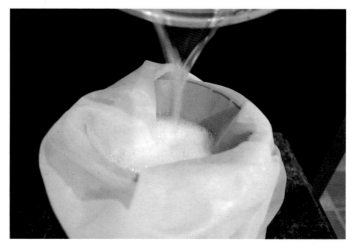

Figure 26.4 Strain through cheesecloth.

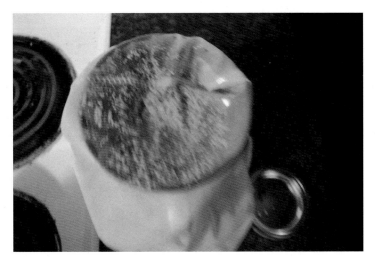

Figure 26.5 Strained milk solids

5. Store in an airtight container.

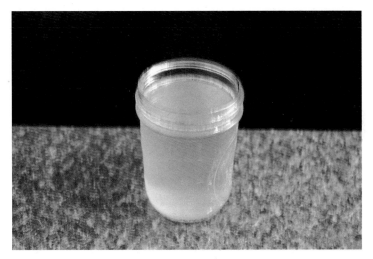

Figure 26.6 Beautiful clarified butter

Yield:
1 pound butter will fill a pint mason jar

Project 27:

Garbage Can Cold Smoker

Being able to smoke foods for preservation was a key pioneer ability. Being able to smoke foods for taste is a prime hobby for many modern men. There is a difference in the times and levels of smoking, but the process is the same—low temperature smoking chambers that surround the meat in smoke from either a small or a separate fire.

You can buy smokers, but they typically cost more than my wife will let me spend on a "grill." This means if I want one I would have to make it. This project cost less than $75, when a store bought smoker of this size would be more than $300 to $400.

I happened to have a small kettle-type grill lying around. I had broken it and then welded the leg back, but it was not too wobbly for tailgating, so I don't use it anymore.

Using the old grill as a base, I was able to fabricate a large capacity smoker that works very well for my home use. If you take this project as a guide, I am sure you can adapt it to whatever scrap you have around and reduce your cost significantly.

Materials:
- Small kettle-type grill
- *Clean* (new) 50-gallon galvanized trash can (or, better yet, a 30- or 50-gallon food safe metal drum)
- Steel flexible hose (*not* Mylar dryer vent)
- 2 metal duct "starters"
- 2 large hose clamps
- 2 (or 3) metal grill grates
- Assorted nuts, bolts, and rivets
- Optional metal duct tape (not grey fabric duck tape)

Tools:

- Drill
- Wrenches/rachet
- Screwdriver
- Measuring tape
- Tin snips
- Rivet gun

Procedure:

1. Cut a hole in the top half of the old grill and an equal-sized hole in the side of the garbage can a couple inches from the bottom. These holes have the same inner diameter as the starters. The starters are round ducts that have tabs cut along one side. These tabs can be pulled out 90 degrees to form a flange to attach to a square duct. Then a round duct can be pushed over the starter.

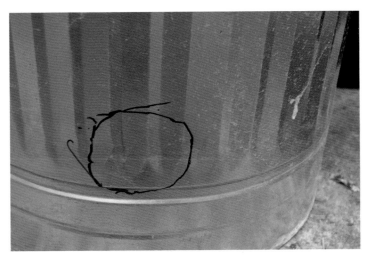

Figure 27.1 Mark a circle the size of the inside of your starter tap and cut it out.

2. I pulled out the tabs and attached the starter tabs to both the grill and the can (one each).

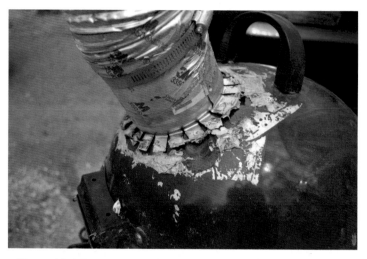

Figure 27.2 Tabs are pulled out and a couple riveted in place.

3. I then loosened one hose clamp, pushed it on one end of the flexible duct, and then pressed the duct over the starter tab. I tightened the clamp over the hose and used the metal tape to make the connection airtight (I found this to not be necessary).

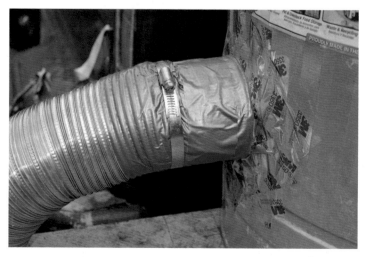

Figure 27.3 Metal hose is attached to starter.

4. Before connecting the hose to the garbage can, you need to attach the smoker grates to the can. Otherwise you will fight with the hose and grill body as you turn the can around to drill the holes.
5. Mark four equidistant holes about halfway up the can.
6. Drill out the holes and put a stainless steel bolt in each hole. (If you were to run string through the holes, the string would form an "X" in the center of the can.) By inserting the bolt and then tightening a nut on the inside, each bolt will form a stop to hold the bracket.

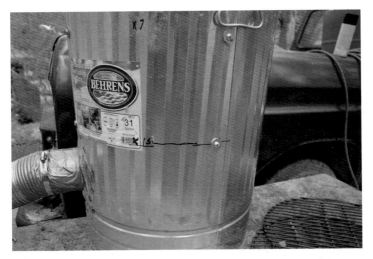

Figure 27.4 To ensure level grates, I marked holes 7 inches from the top lip of the can, and another set 15 inches from the top.

7. I did the same thing about three-quarters way up the can—this forms the upper grill.

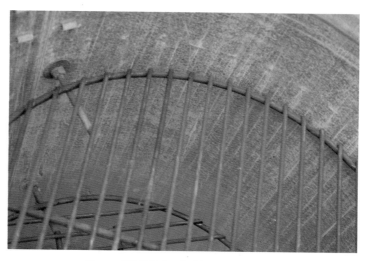

Figure 27.5 Bolts hold up the grate.

8. I took the grates out (leaving the bolts) and attached the hose coming from the grill to the can.

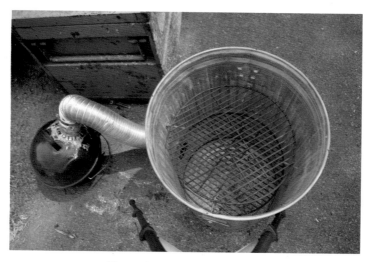

Figure 27.6 Finished smoker

9. Now that the hose is attached, usage is simple: Light a fire in the grill.

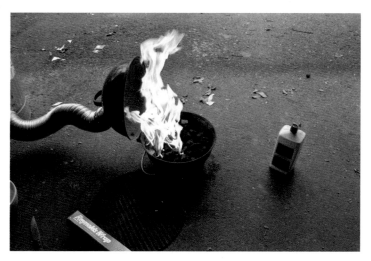

Figure 27.7 Light a fire.

10. Make a bowl out of heavy duty aluminum foil and fill with wood chips (this works best if they are soaked in water for 30 minutes to an hour before usage).

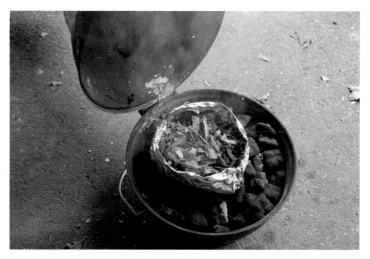

Figure 27.8 Bowl of wet chips

11. Place bowl on the grill grate and close the grill.
12. Smoke will soon leave the grill, travel down the hose, and start to fill the garbage can.
13. Place whatever food you want to smoke on the grill gates in the can.

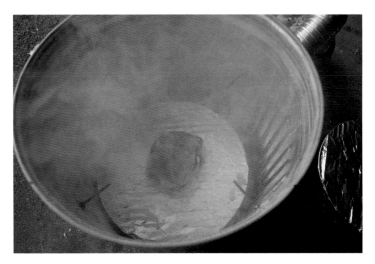

Figure 27.9 Smoking bacon

14. Put the lid on the can and wait as long as it takes to get the level of smoke you desire.

Note:

This is a cold smoke and will not *cook* the meat, so you must use curing salt or other means to protect your food against food-borne illness.

The can is galvanized, and when galvanized metal is heated to over 200°F, the zinc will burn off and the fumes will give you an extreme headache. However, cold smoking stays under 200°F, so it should not be a problem. If you are worried about zinc poisoning, you can simply heat the can up to 300°F to ensure the zinc is burned off before using.

Project 28:
Link Sausage

Sausage is a traditional way to extend the storage life of fresh meat. The traditional skills needed to butcher and preserve meat will serve a prepper well in the event of a catastrophic disaster.

Besides being a useful "End of The World as We Know It" skill, sausage making is a valuable skill for the home cook. The taste of fresh sausage is incomparable to sausage made in an unknown meat processing plant, and the ingredients are of a much higher quality without a large increase in cost.

The only issues with home sausage making is keeping the area extremely clean and keeping the meat cold while working.

In this project, we are going to make an Italian sausage using a homemade spice recipe. It is also very simple to purchase premade mixes, if you prefer.

The most difficult part of the process is encasing the meat in links, and it is an optional step. At the most basic, sausage making involves mixing spices in ground meat—and almost anyone can do that.

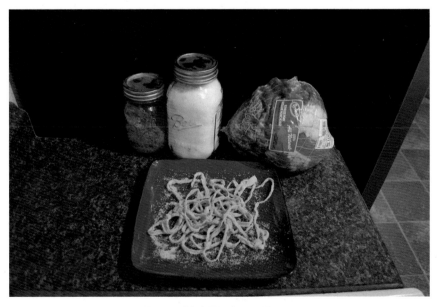

Figure 28.1 The ingredients

Spice mix

Ingredients:

- 1 teaspoon sea salt
- 1 tablespoon fennel seeds, ground
- 1 tablespoon ground sage
- 1 tablespoon garlic powder
- 1 tablespoon onion powder
- ¼ teaspoon white pepper (or 1 teaspoon black pepper)
- 2 teaspoons dried parsley (optional)

Procedure:

1. Combine all ingredients in a mixing bowl.
2. Store in an airtight container for up to 6 months.

Italian Sausage

Ingredients:

- 5 pounds pork shoulder (with fat intact)
- 1 cup spice mix
- 3 tablespoons pink curing salt
- 3 cups water
- Casing (I used natural casings, but collagen casings work fine too.)

Equipment:

- Sharp knife and cutting board
- 2 bowls
- Meat grinder
- Measuring cup
- Sausage stuffer
- Cookie sheet
- Cold smoker

Procedure:

1. The meat needs to be extremely cold (but not frozen). By grinding, you increase the surface area for bacteria contamination, so everything must be kept clean and the meat cold enough to hurt your hands after long exposure in order to reduce the risk of food-borne illnesses.
2. To reduce "smearing" when grinding, trim all silverskin and fat from your pork shoulder. Discard silverskin and cube the fat.

3. Cube the shoulder into 1-inch chunks.

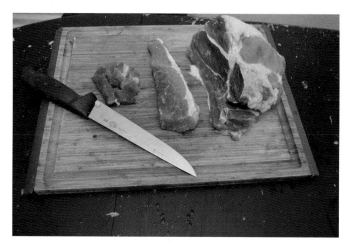

Figure 28.2 Trim into chunks.

4. Grind both the chunks of meat and fat. If the grinder stops putting out nice streams of ground meat and instead jams up and "smushes" out a paste, then the grinder has "smeared" and the easiest way to fix it is to take the grinder apart and clean it.

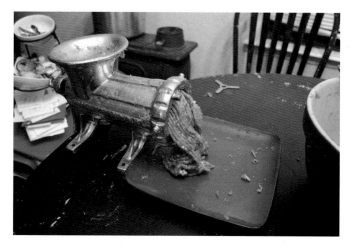

Figure 28.3 Nice ribbons of fresh ground meat come out.

5. Put into a covered container or top the bowl with plastic wrap and put the sausage mixture into the freezer for at least 30 minutes and no more than an hour.

6. Remove the ground fat/meat mix and pour on your spice mix as well as the curing salt. You need at least 2 grams of salt per 100 grams of meat—any more than 3 or 4 percent salt will really mess up your sausage. Many people dislike the nitrates in pink salt, but it is essential in smoked or cured sausage as the conditions in the smoker are perfect for incubating botulism and other biological nasties.

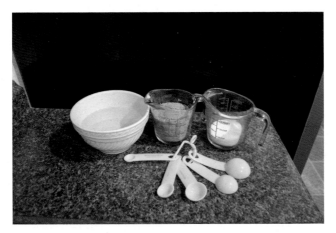

Figure 28.4 Add spices, salt cure, and water.

7. Mix in one cup of water (it helps with holding the meat together as it goes into the cases). In traditional Italian sausages you would use ¾ cup white wine and ¼ cup white wine vinegar, but this method is simpler.
8. Regrind the mix to incorporate the spices.

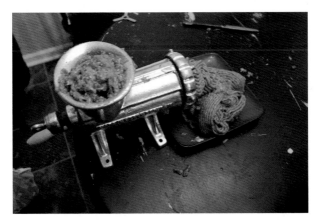

Figure 28.5 Regrind mix.

9. Put your mix back in the cooler to chill for an hour.
10. While your mix is chilling, open your package of casings, wash off any packing salt, and let set in warm water for about an hour.
11. Open the tip of your casing, slide it over the moistened end of your sausage stuffer tube, and then carefully work the casing toward the inside end of the tube bunching it "accordion style"—leave about 3–6 inches hanging loose.

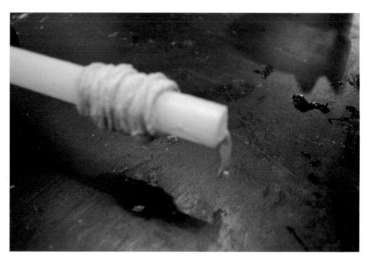

Figure 28.6 Casing is pressed on "accordion style."

12. Insert meat into the stuffer. Start pressing the stuffer down. Air should be the first thing that emerges, which is why you do not tie the casing right off the bat.

13. When the meat starts to come out, use one hand to regulate how fast the casing slips off the tube, and the other to operate the stuffer.

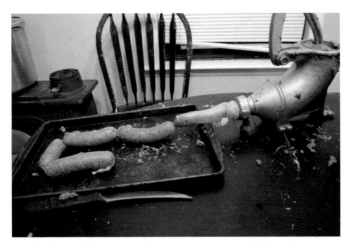

Figure 28.7 Meat coming out of stuffer

14. When the sausage is all in the casings, tie off the one end or use fine butcher's twine.
15. With two hands, pinch off the area that will divide two links. Work the links to force any air bubbles to the ends and spin the links to twist them into separate links. Reverse the direction of spin with each new link. If the first link was turned clockwise, turn the next link counterclockwise when linking so that they don't unravel.

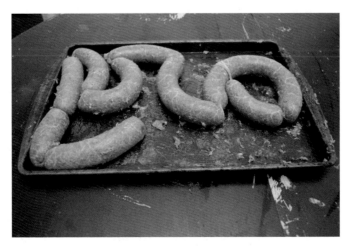

Figure 28.8 Twisted into links

16. Let the sausage rest in the refrigerator overnight so that the meat can set.
17. Let the sausages sit at room temperature for an hour to dry a little before smoking. This gives it a tacky feel that helps the smoke adhere to the sausage.
18. Cold smoke (under 200°F) for a couple hours.

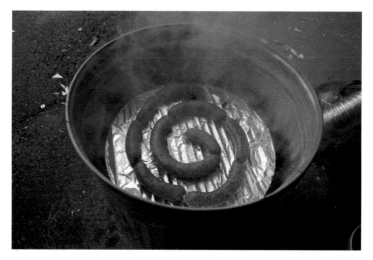

Figure 28.9 Cold smoke for 2 hours.

19. Use within a week or freeze in airtight containers for up to a year.

Yield:
Makes 5 lbs of sausage, or about 15–20 links.

Project 29: Smoked Bacon

Like my first forays into home cheese making, curing bacon used to hold an element of mystery and magic for me. But just like cheese, as soon as I made my first batch of prime home cured and smoked bacon, I was hooked. It is a very simple process and the quality is much better.

This, among all the other projects, is something that the wife says she wants me to repeat. Homemade bacon is easy, tasty, and, depending on where you get your pork from, can be cheaper than store bought bacon.

All you need is a whole pork belly, the curing mix (which I will show you how to make), and a smoker that works in the 150–200°F range.

As with all cooking projects, and especially meat recipes, before you begin you need to clean your work area. You need lots of space and you want whatever your meat touches to be grime free.

The next thing you need to do is to make a dry cure mix. I make mine in large quantities because it stores indefinitely, and it is easier to mix ahead of time.

Dry cure is a mix of non-iodized salt, sugar, and pink salt. Pink salt is normal table salt that has had sodium nitrate added to it, along with a pink die to differentiate it from pure salt. They do this because sodium nitrate is poisonous in large quantities. However, you *must* have pink salt to prevent the growth of botulism spores in the meat. The curing and smoking process is the perfect breeding ground for bacteria, and the nitrate keeps the bacteria from growing. However, by mixing pink salt with other ingredients, we keep the nitrate levels as low as reasonably achievable and still get its benefits.

First, let's start with the dry cure:

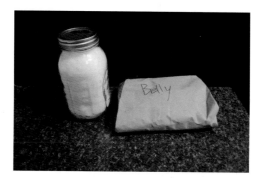

Figure 29.1 The ingredients

Ingredients:

- 1 lb kosher salt
- 8 oz sugar
- 10 teaspoons pink curing salt

I normally double this so that I can use a 1 pound bag of sugar.

Procedure:

- Mix the three ingredients and store in an airtight jar.

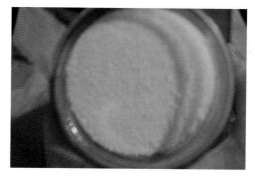

Figure 29.2 Pink salt

It will last pretty much forever and can be used in many other cured meats. Now that you have the pink salt, let's begin making your bacon.

Ingredients:

- Pork belly
- Curing salt
- Optionally, brown sugar, molasses, coffee grounds, and spices can be used to flavor your bacon, but in this project I stayed simple and just threw on some maple syrup right before smoking.

Tools:

- Tongs to maneuver the bacon
- Large pot or 3-gallon freezer bags
- Smoker
- Wood chips (mild hardwood chips like apple seem to work best)
- Optionally, latex gloves are nice.

Procedure:

1. Obtain a whole, raw pork belly. The better quality meat, the better your bacon.

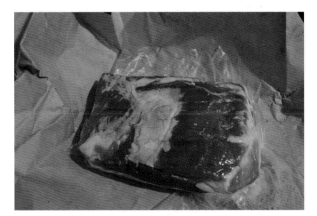

Figure 29.3 Good quality pork belly

2. You can remove the skin (which is great for making cracklings), or leave it on. I have read differing arguments on various sites and books on which is better, and I have tried both. Skin on is easier, but can cause the bacon

to curve as it cures, due to the difference in permeability. Skin off is harder, but you end up with skin to make cracklings.

3. Trim the edges of the belly so they are square-shaped with a clean cut.
4. Spread approximately ⅛ cup of the dry-cure mix out and dredge one side of the belly in it until you have a nice even coating.

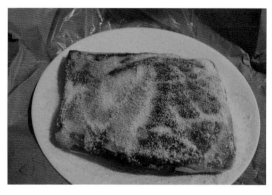

Figure 29.4 Cover with cure.

5. Pour on another ⅛ cup of the mix and do the same to the other side and the edges.
6. Rub it in with your (gloved) hands.
7. If you want to use spices such as molasses, honey, brown sugar, or coffee grounds, drizzle on an even coat on both sides.
8. Carefully slide the belly into a ziplock bag. Alternatively, you don't have to use a bag if you place it in a large nonreactive bowl or dish; just be aware that the salt will pull out a lot of moisture and the bag keeps everything from turning into a mess.

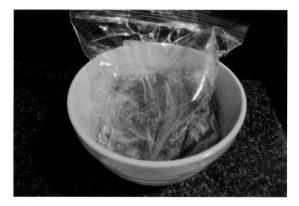

Figure 29.5 A ziplock bag reduces mess.

9. Every 48 hours, flip the belly over. This helps evenly distribute the brine for a better cure.
10. Different bellies will give up more water than others. Expect anywhere from ½ cup to almost 2 cups. In my experience, bellies with the skin attached will be wetter than skinless ones.
11. Bacon will take 7–10 days to cure, depending on size, thickness, etc. They are done curing when the meat is no longer squishy and springy like raw meat. It will have a consistency close to but with slightly more give than silly putty.

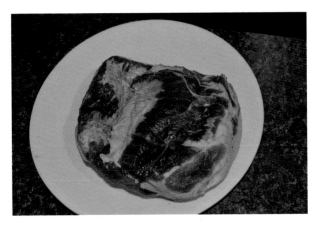

Figure 29.6 The cured bacon is much darker and more solid feeling than raw pork belly.

12. When the belly is done curing, rinse it thoroughly in the sink and pat it dry with paper towels. You want to remove as much of the remaining cure from the meat as possible. I did not do this very well the first time and ended up with an extremely salty product.
13. The night before smoking, leave the belly sitting in the fridge uncovered for 12–24 hours. This will let the meat form a tacky pellicle that will help it absorb the smoke.
14. Before smoking, let the pork belly warm to room temperature.
15. Light your smoker. You want a cooking chamber temperature between 150–200°F. Any hotter than 200°F and you'll be roasting the bellies, not smoking them.
16. I usually smoke with applewood chips. You can use whatever hardwood you want, but softwoods like pine have a high resin content that will deposit tar on your bacon.

17. Smoke the bellies until they reach an internal temperature of 150°F.
18. Follow all safety protocols for your smoker, as well as all local regulations.
19. Wrap the bacon slab in foil and let it rest at room temperature for an hour or so before moving it back to the fridge.

Yield:

Yield depends on the size of the pork belly and the thickness of your slices.

Notes:

Once it's thoroughly chilled, it will be much easier to slice. I have a small deli slicer I use when processing a slab of bacon like this and set it to take nice thick slices, about ⅛ inch or so. If you don't have a slicer, use your longest, sharpest carving knife and mind your fingers!

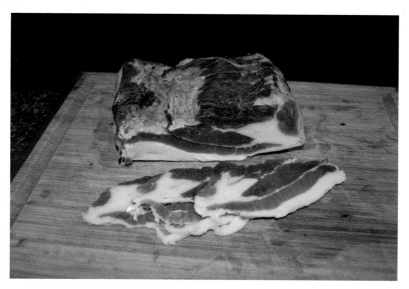

Figure 29.7 Sliced bacon

If stored in an airtight container, the sliced bacon should keep for a good 3–4 weeks in the fridge. Vacuum sealed and frozen will give it an even longer shelf life.

Project 30:
Pressure Canning Bacon

Making your own bacon is really easy, and the whole idea of curing bacon is to increase the storage life of pork in order to get through the winter with meat to eat. So, strictly speaking, canning bacon should be redundant.

Unfortunately, bacon is not made with a view toward food preservation anymore—the salt content is not as high as it should be for long-term storage. This means that while a slab of "Big Dave's Famous Bacon" from Project 29 might easily last 6 months in the fridge, the pre-sliced vacuum sealed grocery store variety may need some help . . .

Another reason you may want to can your bacon is if you find a good deal on bacon end pieces. Since pork belly is not perfectly flat and square, the food processor ends up with bits and pieces of bacon trimming that they box up and sell in bulk.

Bacon end pieces are a lot cheaper, and since canned bacon won't get crispy, I did not want to "waste" strips. This bacon is perfect for flavoring beans or greens. This technique is perfect for that because you can just pull out the can and dump it in a large pot right in with the beans.

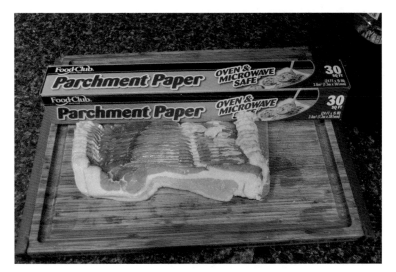

Figure 30.1 The ingredients

Ingredients:

- Bacon

Materials/Tools:

- Parchment paper (if you are canning slices)
- Scissors
- Yardstick
- Sterile wide-mouth quart mason jar, lids and rings (1 per pound of sliced bacon)
- Canning tongs
- Pressure canner

Procedure for End Pieces:

It's pretty simple: divide your end pieces, stuff them raw into your canning jars (bacon is packed both dry and raw), then process your jars at 10 pounds for 90 minutes.

Procedure for Slices:

1. Roll out the paper to about two feet in length.
2. Lay slices of bacon on the paper, as close as you can to each other without overlapping. A quart jar will hold a pound of bacon, but the actual number of slices will depend on the thickness of the cut.

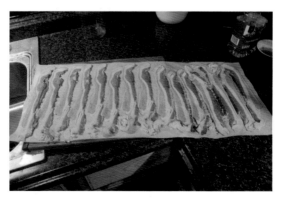

Figure 30.2 Lay bacon on paper without any overlap.

3. Cut the paper at the end of the line of bacon. Don't leave a "tail" of paper. Now lay another layer of paper over the top and trim to the same length as the lower layer of paper.

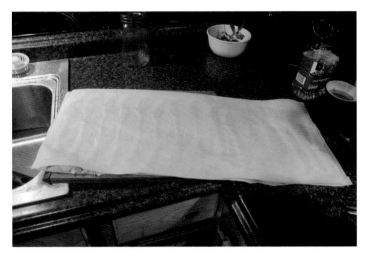

Figure 30.3 Cover with more paper.

4. Place another sheet of parchment paper over the bacon, making a "bacon paper sandwich."
5. Lay a yardstick lengthwise across the center of the bacon and use it as a guide to fold the bacon slices in half over themselves.

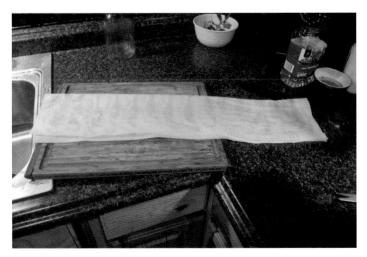

Figure 30.4 Fold in half.

6. Roll the bacon sandwich up tightly. You need to take care that the package is small enough to fit in your jar.

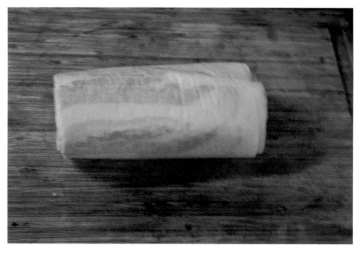

Figure 30.5 Roll tightly.

7. Slip the package into the jar. I used to not care what orientation the bacon went in, but I learned a really cool tip from Kellene Bishop, the Preparedness Pro: if you place the package open end down, the bacon grease will drip into the bottom of the jar, causing less mess and an easier time getting to the fat to reuse it later. (This shows why talking to others and learning by doing is quite helpful, because I have never thought of this and I have canned a good amount of bacon.)

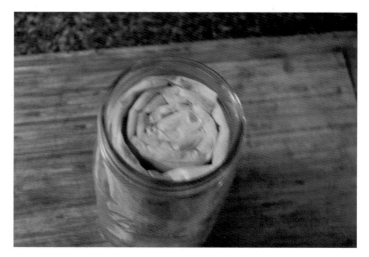

Figure 30.6 Slip into jar, open end down.

8. Once the package is fit nicely inside the jar, put on the lid and process it in a pressure canner at 10 pounds of pressure for 90 minutes. Remember that bacon is dry packed raw, so do not add water or anything else to your bacon.

Project 31: Corned Beef

This is another extremely simple process that is useful, but that most people think is difficult. If you make your own corned beef, you can customize it to your particular tastes, and you will have also learned another way to help preserve your meat a little longer. If you add this recipe to the project on homemade sauerkraut later in the book, you will have the makings of a fine meal . . .

Corning comes from the worn "corn"—meaning "grain," as in grain of salt. Any cut of meat can be corned, but the process works best with the tougher (and cheaper) cuts like brisket. At its most basic, all you really need is meat, salt, and water; but now that sodium nitrate is easily available, it should be used to prevent food-borne illness.

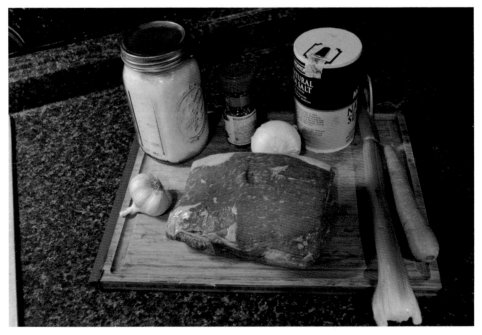

Figure 31.1 The ingredients

Ingredients:

- 5-pound beef brisket
- 1 ½ cups kosher salt
- 4 teaspoons pink salt (sodium nitrite)
- 1 gallon of water
- ½ cup sugar

Optional:

- 3 cloves garlic, minced
- 4 tablespoons pickling spice*
- 1 carrot, peeled and roughly chopped
- 1 medium onion, peeled and cut in two
- 1 celery stalk, roughly chopped

Equipment:

- Large pot
- Measuring cups
- Plate
- Food safe weight (like a large unopened food can)

Procedure:

1. Combine 1 gallon of water with salt, sugar, sodium nitrite, garlic, and 2 tablespoons pickling spice.
2. Bring to a simmer, stirring until salt and sugar are dissolved.
3. Remove from heat and let cool to room temperature.
4. Refrigerate until chilled.

5. Place brisket in brine, weighted with a plate to keep it submerged, and cover. Refrigerate for 5 days.

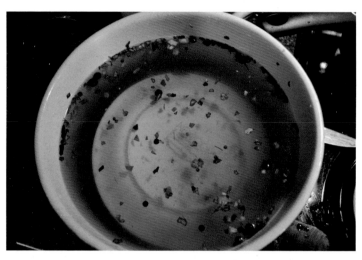

Figure 31.2 Beef is held underwater by the weight of a plate.

If you are going to make pastrami, skip to the bonus section. Otherwise keep reading to learn how to cook the corned beef.

6. Remove brisket from brine and rinse thoroughly.
7. Place in a pot just large enough to hold it. Cover with water and add remaining pickling spice, carrot, onion, and celery.

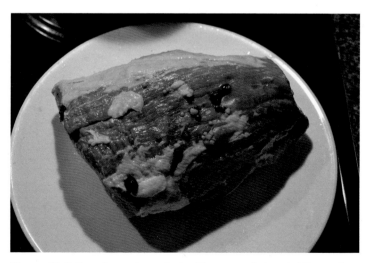

Figure 31.3 Cured meat covered with some of the pickling spice.

8. Bring to a boil over high heat, reduce heat to low, and cover.
9. Simmer gently until brisket is fork-tender, about 3 hours, adding water if needed to cover brisket.
10. Keep warm until ready to serve.

Meat can be refrigerated for several days in cooking liquid.

Yield:
   8–10 servings

Pickling Spice

Ingredients:

- 2 tablespoons black peppercorns
- 2 tablespoons mustard seeds
- 2 tablespoons coriander seeds
- 2 tablespoons hot red pepper flakes
- 2 tablespoons allspice berries
- 1 tablespoon ground mace
- 2 small cinnamon sticks, crushed or broken into pieces
- 2 to 4 bay leaves, crumbled
- 2 tablespoons whole cloves
- 1 tablespoon ground ginger

Procedure:

1. Combine peppercorns, mustard seeds, and coriander seeds in a small dry pan.
2. Place over medium heat and stir until fragrant, being careful not to burn them; keep lid handy in case seeds pop.
3. Crack peppercorns and seeds in mortar and pestle or with the side of a knife on cutting board.
4. Combine with other spices and mix. Store in tightly sealed plastic or glass container.

Bonus Project: Pastrami

If you have a smoker (you should if you have been following along) and if you have some corned beef, you may find that pastrami is simply corned beef smoked with a special rub.

Because smoke also enhances the storage life of meat, you may want to try your hand at making this delicious bonus recipe.

Ingredients:

- 5-pound corned beef
- 1 gallon of water
- 1 cup of cooking oil

Optional rub (purists would say that without the rub it is not pastrami—but I like it just as well without as I do with a traditional rub)

- 4 tablespoons fresh coarsely ground black pepper
- 2 tablespoons coriander powder
- 1 teaspoon mustard powder
- 1 tablespoon brown sugar
- 1 tablespoon paprika
- 2 teaspoons garlic powder
- 2 teaspoons onion powder

Equipment:

- Large pot
- Smoker
- Smoker fuel and smoker wood for at least 4 but preferably 12 hours
- Aluminum foil

Procedure:

1. Rinse off and then soak the corned beef in fresh water for at least 8 hours; otherwise you will have a *very* salty hunk of beef.

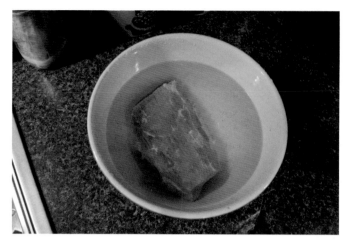

Figure 31.4 Soaking beef removes salt.

2. Mix the *optional* (but recommended) spice mix. It is not true pastrami without the rub.
3. Coat the meat in a thin layer of cooking oil and rub the spice mix in the meat at approximately 4 tablespoons of mix per square foot of meat.
4. Chill in fridge for 2 days.
5. Smoke at 190–200°F for at least 4 hours, but you will be much happier if you smoke this pastrami for closer to 12.

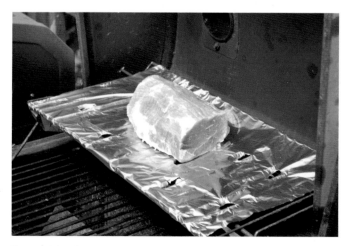

Figure 31.5 Cold smoke for as long as you can stand waiting.

6. Wrap in foil and let chill for 12 hours.
7. Serve by slicing ⅛ inch thick perpendicular to the grain and steaming to 203°F.

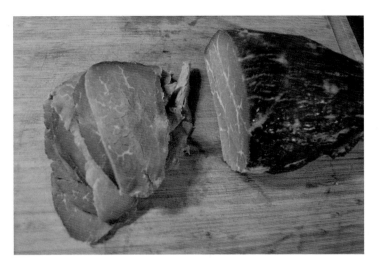

Figure 31.6 Slice, steam, and enjoy.

Yield:
   8–10 servings

Project 32: Sauerkraut

Sauerkraut is a great first fermentation project for kitchen DIY experimentation because it is easy, does not require special equipment, and the results are pretty dependable with little to go wrong.

Since the bacteria that ferments the cabbage is already on it, all you really need to do is combine shredded cabbage with some salt and pack it into a container. This version doesn't even need a crock as we will introduce the concept using mason jars.

Sauerkraut is made by lacto-fermentation. All fruits and vegetables have a strain of bacteria called *Lactobacillus* on their skin, and, when submerged in brine, the bacteria convert sugars into lactic acid. Just like the bacteria in your body, having a large amount of healthy bacteria crowds out and fights dangerous bacteria; this is why lacto-fermentation acts as a natural preservative.

The fermentation process is very reliable and safe, and has been used for centuries to preserve food. Fermented sauerkraut can be kept at cellar temperature (around 55°F) for months, although a refrigerator will work if you don't have a root cellar. In addition to the storage properties, lacto-fermentation has the additional health benefit of being probiotic.

This process is easy and not a lot can go wrong. You may see bubbles, foam, or white scum on the surface of the sauerkraut, but those are all signs of normal, healthy fermentation. Really, as long as you keep the cabbage submerged so it does not mold, it really is foolproof; but like with all home food preservation techniques, trust your senses. If you think it smells or looks bad, toss it and start the process over.

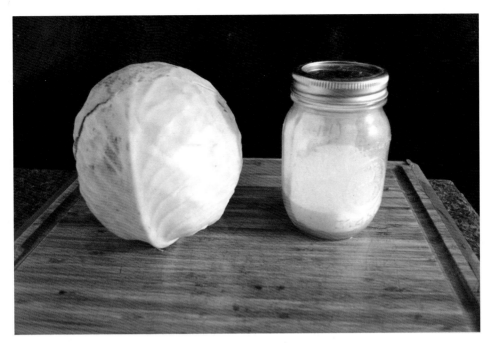

Figure 32.1 The ingredients

Ingredients:

- 1 medium head green cabbage (about 3 pounds)
- 1 ½ tablespoons kosher salt
- 1 tablespoon caraway seeds (optional, for flavor)

Equipment:

- Knife
- Mixing bowl
- Canning funnel
- 2 sterile quart wide-mouth canning jars with lids and rings
- Smaller jelly jar that fits inside the larger mason jar
- Clean weights for weighing the jelly jar down
- Cloth
- Rubber band

Procedure:

1. Clean and sterilize everything.
2. Slice the cabbage.

    a. Save a couple firm outer leaves of the cabbage and reserve for later.

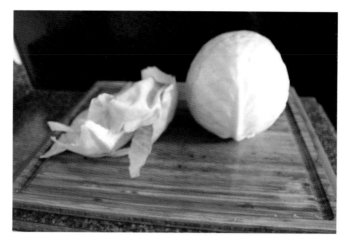

Figure 32.2 Save some leaves for later.

    b. Discard any wilted leaves of the cabbage.
    c. Cut into quarters and trim out the core.
    d. Slice each quarter down its length, making 8 wedges.

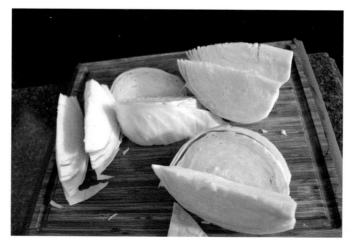

Figure 32.3 Cut head into eighths.

3. Slice each wedge crosswise into very thin ribbons.

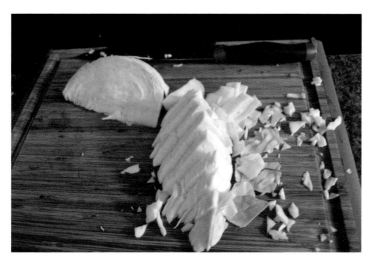

Figure 32.4 Cut sections into thin ribbons.

4. Put the cabbage ribbons into a mixing bowl and sprinkle cabbage with salt.

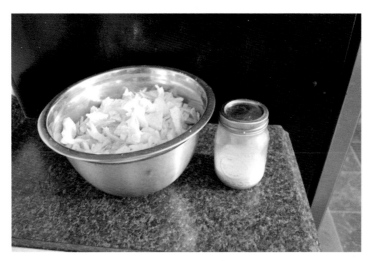

Figure 32.5 Coat with salt.

5. Work the salt into the cabbage by massaging the cabbage with your hands.

   a. You may think you do not have enough salt, but after 5–10 minutes, the cabbage will take on the consistency of coleslaw—watery and limp.

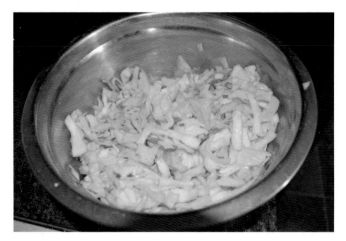

Figure 32.6 Massage until cabbage has wilted and become moist.

6. If you want to flavor your kraut with caraway, mix them in now.
7. Put your canning funnel in the jar and pack your jars with the cabbage. Tamp the limp cabbage in the jar with your fingers.

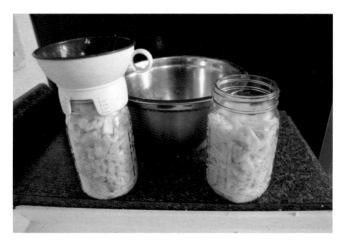

Figure 32.7 Pack tightly.

8. Pour any liquid released by the cabbage while you were massaging it into the jar.

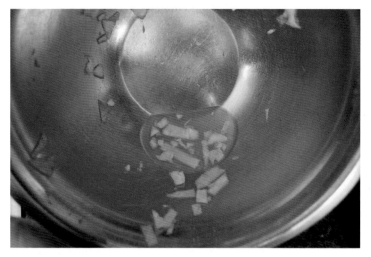

Figure 32.8 Liquid is created by salting cabbage.

9. Place one of the larger outer leaves of the cabbage over the surface of the sliced cabbage. (This keeps the cabbage submerged in its liquid, which prevents the formation of mold.)

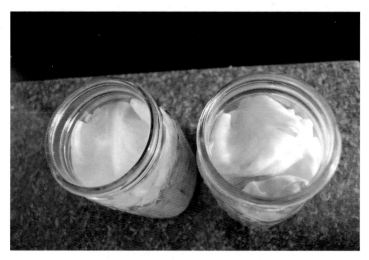

Figure 32.9 Place leaves in top of jar.

10. Once your jars are full, fill your jelly jars with clean rocks or other weights and slide the small jar inside the mouth of the wide-mouth jar. This will push on the cabbage leaf, which will press the sauerkraut under the liquid.

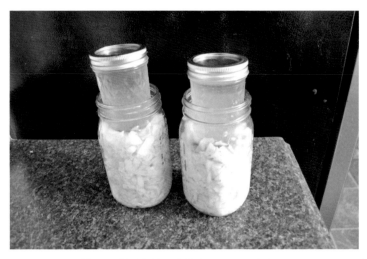

Figure 32.10 Use jelly jars as weights.

11. Cover the mouth of the mason jar with the cloth and secure it with a rubber band. This process needs a little airflow, but not any bugs or dust.

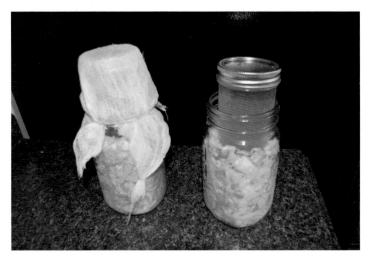

Figure 32.11 Cover with cloth secured by a rubber band.

12. Over the next 24 hours, press down on the jelly jar every couple of hours to compact the cabbage and press out any liquid. Eventually the released moisture will cover the cabbage.

    a. After 24 hours, if the liquid has not risen above the cabbage, dissolve 1 teaspoon of salt in 1 cup of water and add enough to submerge the cabbage.

13. Ferment the cabbage for 3–10 days, keeping the sauerkraut away from direct sunlight and at a cool room temperature, ideally 65–75°F.
14. Check it daily and press it down if the cabbage is floating above the liquid.
15. Start tasting it after 3 days. When the sauerkraut tastes good to you, remove the weight, screw on the cap, and refrigerate.

Yield:
  1–1 ½ quarts

Notes:
  You can water bath can sauerkraut for longer storage outside of refrigeration, but the canning process will kill the good bacteria produced by the fermentation process. Raw pack the sauerkraut to ½ inch of head space and process quarts for 25 minutes.

  To make different-sized batches of sauerkraut, keep same ratio of cabbage to salt and adjust the size of the container. Smaller batches will ferment more quickly and larger batches will take longer.

Project 33:
Kefir

Kefir is a fermented milk drink made with kefir "grains." Kefir grains are a combination of lactic acid bacteria and yeasts in a matrix of proteins, lipids, and sugars. This symbiotic matrix, or SCOBY, forms "grains" that resemble cauliflower. In case you're wondering (and for future projects), "SCOBY" is actually an acronym for "symbiotic culture of bacteria and yeast."

I got started with Kefir when a co-worker told me he inoculated his son's bottles with kefir because his toddler hid his bottles. My buddy assured me that finding a milk bottle under the couch a month or two later was a horrible fate, but that the kefir kept the milk from rotting into a stinky moldy mess.

I had to try it, and it worked very well. Fortunately, my wife keeps an iron hold on the bottles so while my boy loves throwing his bottles behind the couch, his momma hunts them down (it reminds me of when a young Marine lost his rifle at infantry school and the whole battalion spent 67 hours hunting for it—no, it wasn't me . . .).

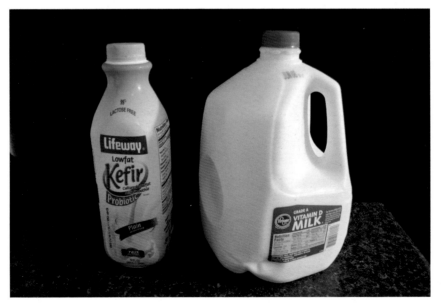

Figure 33.1 The ingredients

Ingredients:

- Kefir grains (easily purchased online and traded for; or you could do what I did and just buy some bottled kefir with live grains at the health food section of the grocery store)
- Milk (any kind but UHP shelf stable box milk)

Equipment:

- Mesh strainer
- Glass or plastic bowl
- Rubber spatula or wooden spoon
- Mason jars

Procedure:

1. Put 1–2 tablespoons of kefir grains into a clean pint-sized mason jar. (The more kefir grains you add, the faster the milk will turn to kefir.)

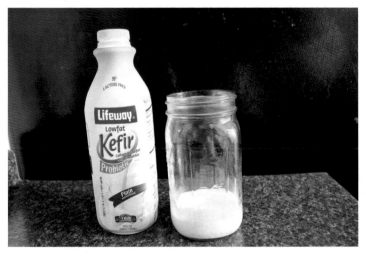

Figure 33.2 Put kefir in the jar.

2. Add milk to ½-inch head space from the top of the jar.

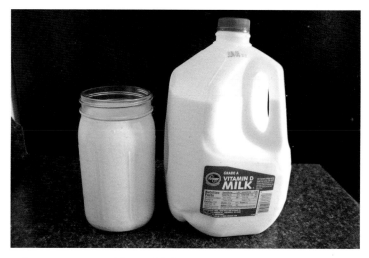

Figure 33.3 Fill with milk.

3. Cover the mason jar with a lid and set it out on the counter for anywhere from 12–36 hours. If you put in the fridge, the SCOBY will go to sleep.

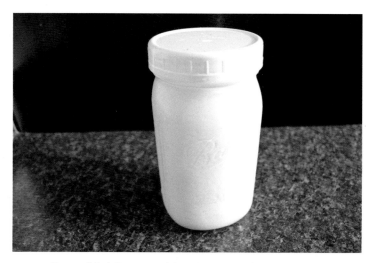

Figure 33.4 Cover and let sit at room temperature.

4. You will know when it is done, as the milk will look thick and clumpy. Like yogurt, the longer it sets at room temperature, the more tangy it will become, and at some point it will separate into a clear liquid and clumps. If that happens, you have a developed kefir (and you can drink it, but it will be very tart).

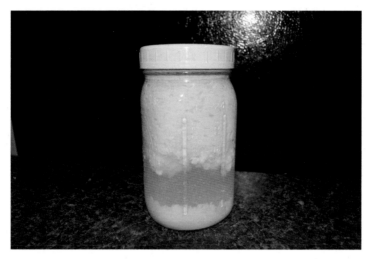

Figure 33.5 Finished kefir

You only need to buy kefir grains once, as you strain the grains out of your cultured milk and reuse them. To do so:

1. Pour the kefir out into a strainer set on top of a glass or plastic bowl.
2. Use a rubber spatula or wooden spoon to gently stir the kefir until all the liquid passes through the mesh and you are left with kefir grains.
3. Store your grains back in a clean mason jar, add some more milk, and start all over again.

Project 34: Kombucha

Kombucha begins as sweet tea, the staple of the south, to which a special SCOBY is added to eat the sugar and transform the sweet tea into a slightly sour carbonated beverage that is low in calories. Some claim that it also has positive health benefits.

Since kombucha is fermented with a live culture, it is full of the probiotic organisms that help your intestines function well. I won't go into all its other purported health benefits because I am not a doctor, and I have not done enough of my own research to be giving health advice. I will mention, however, that while you are researching the health benefits of kombucha, you will also find some who claim it is dangerous since it contains live cultures. I give that about as much credence as the kombucha enthusiasts who say it cures arthritis—there just isn't any evidence. I brew all manner of things on my kitchen counter and find that if you keep your equipment clean and inoculate your food to give the desired bacteria time to grow—they crowd out anything that could get you sick.

In the event that you have cultural, personal, or health reasons to avoid alcohol, you should also note that whenever yeast is used to carbonate a liquid, a by-product of the yeast is alcohol.

Alcohol will form in the carbonation process. It is less than 1 percent and should not get you drunk, but it is also enough to activate cultural taboos in some groups.

This may look complicated, but it really isn't. It's just a more controlled method to get the same result I get if I leave tea glass on the workbench and forget it for a few weeks . . .

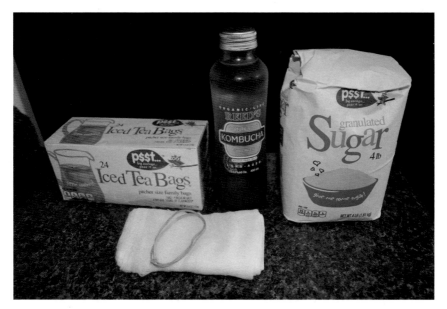

Figure 34.1 The ingredients

Ingredients:

- 3 ½ quarts water
- 1 cup white sugar
- 8 bags black tea (or 2 tablespoons loose tea)
- 2 cups starter tea from last batch of kombucha or store-bought (unpasteurized, neutral-flavored) kombucha

Equipment:

- Stock pot
- 1-gallon glass jar or two 2-quart glass jars (if you don't have large-mouth jars this big, you can use several mason jars)
- Bottles of some type (I just use a clean 2-liter soda bottle)—you need something that can resist pressures formed if you have extra sugar and the yeast keeps working.

Procedure:

1. Make sweet tea. You should not need a recipe for this, but in case you have never brewed tea, here you go:

    a. Bring the water to a boil.
    b. Remove from heat and stir in the sugar to dissolve.
    c. Drop in the tea and allow it to steep until the water has cooled.
    d. Depending on the size of your pot, this will take a few hours.

2. Stir in the starter tea.

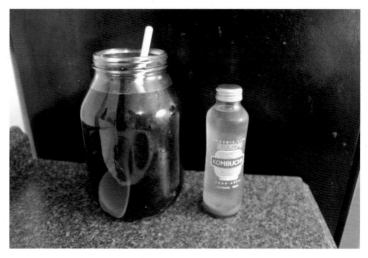

Figure 34.2 Stir in kombucha starter.

3. Transfer to jars and add the SCOBY.

4. Cover the mouth of the jar with a few layers of cheesecloth or paper towels secured with a rubber band.

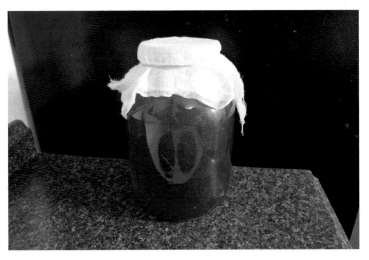

Figure 34.3 Cover and let sit at room temperature.

5. Ferment for 7–10 days. Keep the jar at room temperature, out of direct sunlight, and where it won't get disturbed.

    a. Scoby is a living organism (more accurately, a collection of organisms living symbiotically), so it's not unusual for it to do weird things like float sideways or form brown stringy bits floating beneath the main disk of scoby.

    b. Sediment will collect at the bottom of your jar and, due to the yeast, it may create bubbles. This is all normal and the reason why I don't let my wife see me make it (or she would not drink it).

6. After 7 days, you can taste it daily to find the perfect balance of sweetness and tartness. When it gets the way you want it, bottle it. If it's kept at room temperature it will continue to lose sweetness and gain tartness until the yeast eats all the sugar.

7. If you want to make more, you can recycle the Scoby and begin a new batch. With clean hands, gently lift the Scoby out of the bottle and place it in a new batch of tea. You can even break it up and use it to make several batches (or gift a piece to a friend).

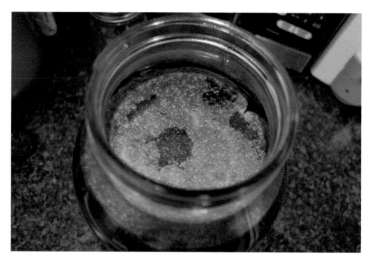

Figure 34.4 Healthy Scoby floats.

8. Bottle the finished kombucha.
9. Refrigerate the kombucha and drink within the month.

Yield:
3 quarts of finished tea

Notes:
To increase or decrease the amount of kombucha you make, maintain the basic ratio of 1 cup of sugar, 8 bags of tea, and 2 cups starter tea per gallon batch. One scoby will ferment any size batch, though larger batches may take longer.

Kombucha will smell progressively more vinegary as brewing progresses. If it starts to smell cheesy, rotten, or otherwise unpleasant, discard the liquid and begin again with fresh tea.

If you do see signs of mold, discard both the scoby and the liquid and begin again with new ingredients.

Project 35:
Crock Pot Yogurt

Homemade yogurt is a simple thing to make. It is believed that the first yogurt was accidently discovered when Mongol warriors drank curdled milk stored in hide wine cloths hung next to the saddles of their warhorses.

While the original curdled milk does not sound appetizing, this yogurt is a great use of extra milk, and it can be used in all manner of homestead recipes.

This recipe is extremely simple and uses equipment that almost everyone has.

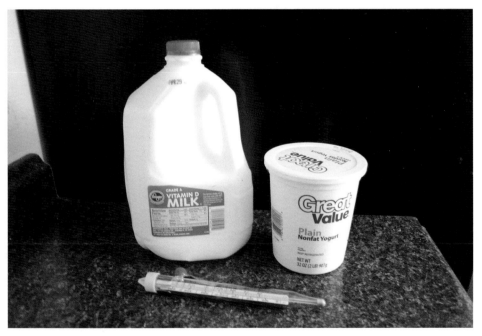

Figure 35.1 The ingredients

Ingredients:

- One gallon milk
- 2 tablespoons plain yogurt (active culture works best)

Equipment:

- Crock pot
- Thermometer
- Measuring cup
- Spoon
- Cheesecloth or filtering bag

Procedure:

1. Place the gallon of milk into the crock pot and heat slowly to between 180–190°F. It is vital to heat the milk to at least 180°F.

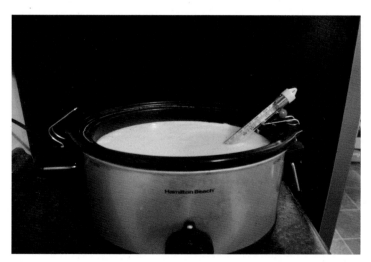

Figure 35.2 Heat to at least 180°F.

2. Allow the milk to cool down naturally to 110°F. This will take about 3 ½–4 hours. It is critical that you catch the milk at 110°F. I check every 10–15 minutes until the temperature is around 125–130°F, then every couple minutes until it gets to the perfect 110°F.

3. If you are using non-homogenized or raw milk there will be a skin that has formed on the top of the milk. If you do not spoon it all off it will turn into hard flakes that are quite unappetizing.

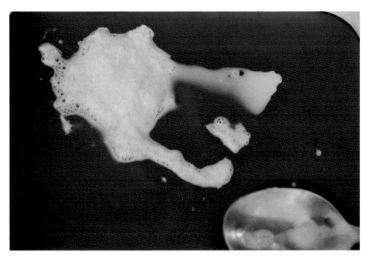

Figure 35.3 Milk skin will form on non-homogenized milk.

4. Remove about 1 cup of warm milk into a separate cup or small bowl. Add 2 tablespoons of starter yogurt to the cup of milk.
5. Gently stir the starter yogurt into the cup of milk to inoculate it.

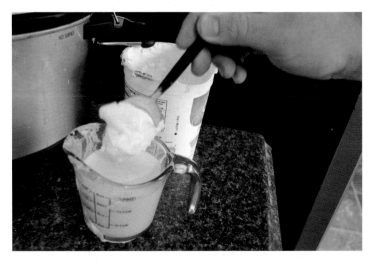

Figure 35.4 Inoculating milk with thermophilic cultures.

6. Pour the inoculated milk into the crock pot and stir in gently going from side to side. Do not stir in circles; use a careful and slow up and down lifting motion moving across the length of the crock. This keeps unwanted bacteria or yeast from being incorporated into the milk.

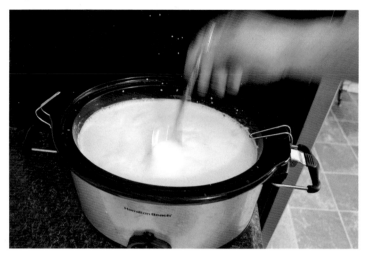

Figure 35.5 Gently whisk in inoculated milk.

7. Lift the covered crock out of its base, wrap it in a blanket and place it into a cool oven. Leave it undisturbed overnight or for about 10–12 hours. If you open the oven door you may have a yogurt failure.

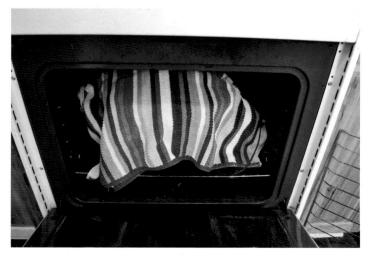

Figure 35.6 Crock is covered with blanket.

8. The yogurt will separate and leave some whey. You need to filter this out. I prefer to use a beer making wort bag, but butter muslin or very thickly woven cheesecloth in a colander would also work. The longer you drain the whey, the thicker the yogurt. This is the difference between plain and Greek yogurt.

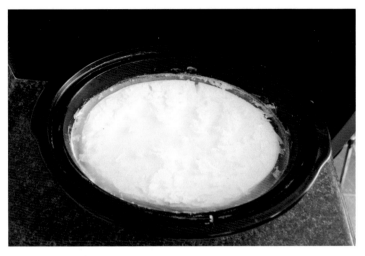

Figure 35.7 Yogurt and whey

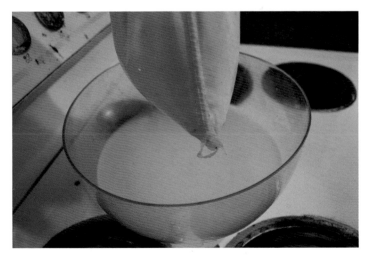

Figure 35.8 Drain the yogurt.

9. If you save some to use as a starter culture, you will never need to purchase yogurt again.

Yield:
Approximately one pound of yogurt per gallon of milk

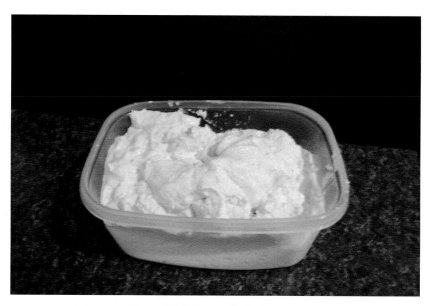

Figure 35.9 One pound of yogurt

Notes:
If you prefer a tart yogurt you can leave this yogurt out on the counter for up to 24 hours. The longer it is left out (up to 24 hours maximum) the tarter it will become.

This is also known as a mesophilic (heat loving) culture and it can be used to make some cheeses. I like to freeze this in an ice cube mold and store in the freezer for future use.

Bonus Project: Mason Jar Oatmeal

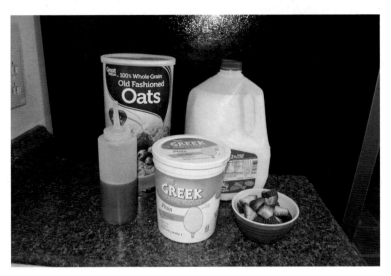

Figure 35.10 The ingredients

Ingredients:

- ¼ cup uncooked oatmeal
- ¼ cup yogurt
- ⅓ cup milk
- Honey optional
- Fruit optional
- 2 teaspoons chia seeds optional

Procedure:

1. Dump oatmeal, yogurt, milk, chia seeds, fruit, and honey to taste into mason jar.

2. Mix well and place lid on jar.

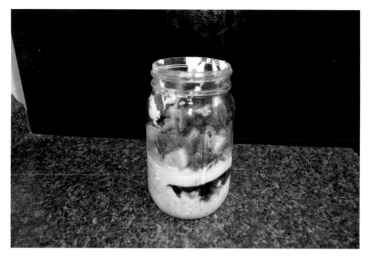

Figure 35.11 Mix ingredients well.

3. Refrigerate overnight.
4. Enjoy.

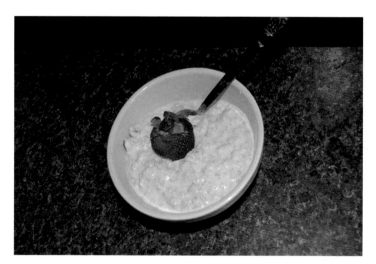

Figure 35.12 Enjoy an easy breakfast.

Yield:
A hearty breakfast for one, or a good breakfast for two

Project 36: Hot Pepper Joint Cream

As a former correctional officer and a current security guard trainer, I have a good bit of experience with capsaicin, which is the component in hot peppers that gives them their heat.

Capsaicin is an inflammatory that makes your eyes and mucus membranes swell shut, your eyes water, and your face feel on fire when it is sprayed on you, so you may wonder why someone would want to put it in a joint cream.

The reason capsaicin is put in over-the-counter pain cream for arthritis, sore muscles, shingles, and psoriasis is that capsaicin overwhelms the nerves and depletes substance P (which is one of the neurotransmitters for pain and heat).

A less scientific reason (but something I have experienced) is that exposure to capsaicin releases endorphins in your body. I always feel better after being sprayed with pepper spray or after eating hot peppers when the heat subsides.

This cream is a great project for preppers as it gives you a good pain relief cream that works when stores may be closed. I like it because I can control the quality of the ingredients, and I feel better when I can use it to treat loved ones because I feel like I took a more active role in reducing their pain.

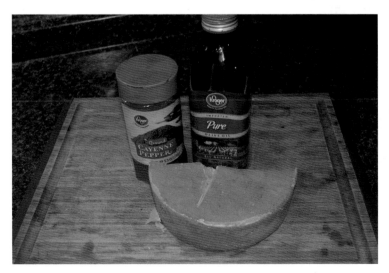

Figure 36.1 The ingredients

Ingredients:

- 3 tablespoons of cayenne powder
- 1 cup of olive oil (or any other oil like grapeseed, almond, or jojoba)
- ½ cup of grated beeswax

Equipment:

- A double boiler
- A glass jar with a tightly fitting lid

Procedure:

1. Mix together 3 tablespoons of cayenne powder with 1 cup of your oil of choice.
2. Heat in a double boiler for 5–10 minutes over medium heat.

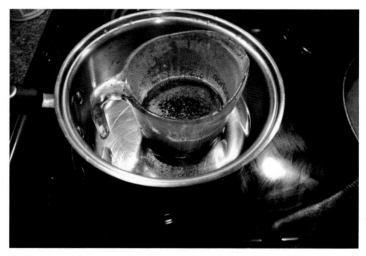

Figure 36.2 Heat oil and pepper in a double boiler.

3. Stir in a ½ cup of grated beeswax and continue to stir until it has melted completely.

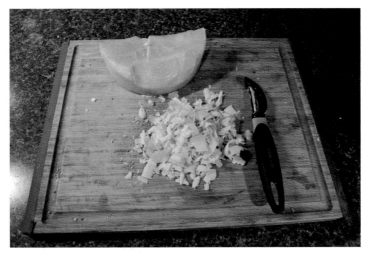

Figure 36.3 An easy way to grate beeswax is to use a potato peeler.

4. Chill the mixture in the refrigerator for 10 minutes, then whisk together.

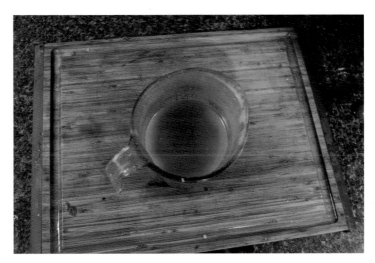

Figure 36.4 Chill and whisk.

5. Chill for another 10–15 minutes, then whip again before putting it in a glass jar with a tightly fitting lid and storing in the refrigerator.

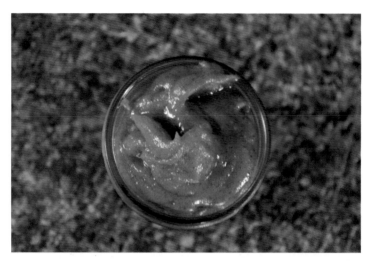

Figure 36.5 Pour into mason jar and use as required.

Notes:

It will keep for 1 ½ weeks. Apply daily as needed for pain.

As this active ingredient is pepper based, it is normal for there to be a burning sensation when first applied. If you have sensitive skin, use with caution.

Always wear gloves when handling hot pepper powder, and avoid any contact with your eyes.

Project 37:
How to Make Homemade Soap

While this is not a food preservation method, I think homemade soap making is a vital project in a book such as this because you cannot cook if you can't get your pots clean.

There is a lot of mystery in home soap making and a lot of techniques out there. Frankly, it can be a little daunting to a beginner. Because of this, I want to introduce you to an easier way to make soap, called the room temperature method. While it may make purists upset, it is easier as you don't need to heat any oils or check any temperatures.

Even though this is an easier method, it does not mean you do not need to be careful or do any research. It still uses lye and it still gets hot so please take the time to read up on the subject and the entire process before you start, rather than reading and performing one line at a time as you go along. Making soap is not like putting together a Lego kit!

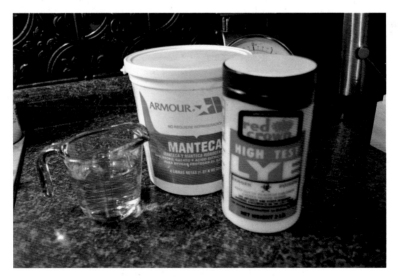

Figure 37.1 The ingredients

Ingredients:

- 1 pound lard (also known as Manteca at the grocery)
- 2.3 ounces lye
- 6.1 ounces distilled water (not tap, filtered, or bottles)

Equipment:

- Nonreactive pot (stainless steel, not aluminum or cast iron)
- Accurate scale
- Whisk (once again nonreactive)
- Soap mold
- Knife
- Towels
- Parchment paper (or thick plastic and tape)
- Immersion blender or electric blender to only be used for soap making (optional, but you will thank me if you get one)

Procedure:

1. Prepare your mold (see below).
2. Weigh out and place lard into your pot.

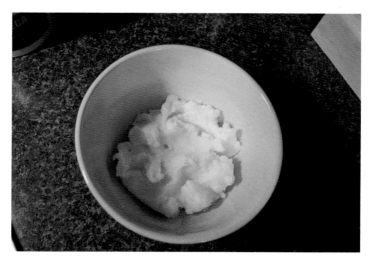

Figure 37.2 Place lard in pot.

3. Prepare your lye solution by weighing out the water and the sodium hydroxide.

4. Slowly pour the sodium hydroxide into the water and gently stir until the crystals dissolve (it will get hot). Always add lye to water and never water to lye, for safety reasons.

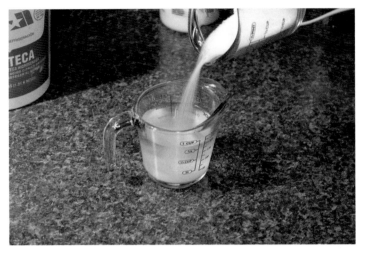

Figure 37.3 Add lye to water—*never* add water to lye.

5. Once the lye solution has become clear, slowly pour the lye water over the hard oils in your pot. The hot solution will melt the oils.

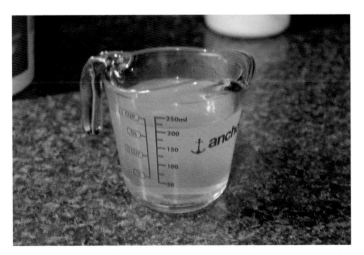

Figure 37.4 Wait for solution to clear (it will be hot).

6. Gently press the oils down into the lye solution with the whisk and slowly stir until the oils are completely melted.

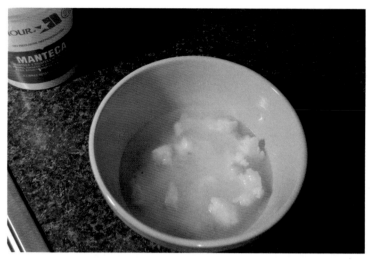

Figure 37.5 Hot lye solution will melt lard.

7. Add the liquid oils to the soap pot and whisk together.
8. Using your stick blender, mix the soap batter in short bursts alternating with hand stirring until the soap reaches a thin trace.

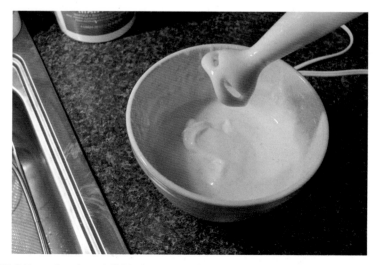

Figure 37.6 Trace is when dribbled soap will leave a trace on the surface of the soap. It is an indicator that the lye and fats are mixed well enough to not separate.

9.   Pour into your prepared soap mold.

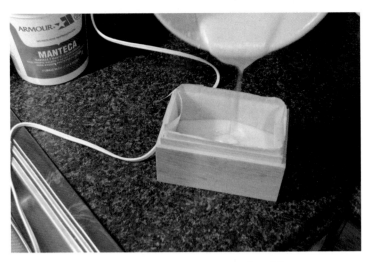

Figure 37.7 Pour into prepared mold.

10. Cover the soap.
11. Wrap and insulate until the soap sets.

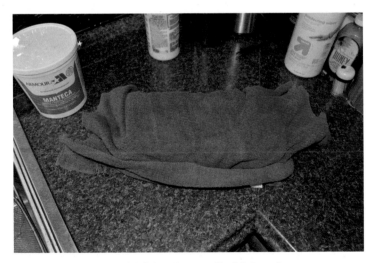

Figure 37.8 Insulate well with towels.

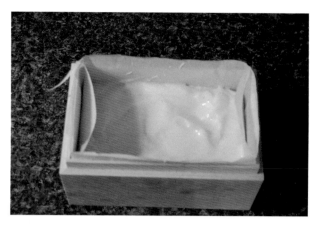

Figure 37.9 Leave alone for 8–12 hours.

12. As soon as the soap has cooled to the touch and is firm enough to handle, you can cut it into bars.

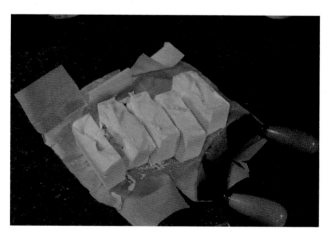

Figure 37.10 Cut and let cure.

13. Cure the soap for 4–6 weeks (this makes the soap more mild and less harsh on your skin).

Yield:
Approximately 1 ½ pounds of soap

Preparing Your Soap Mold

1. Cut a strip of parchment paper twice as long and three times as large as your mold.
2. Place the mold in the center of the paper and mark the paper so you can fold it into thirds lengthways.
3. Place the mold in the center of the folded parchment paper and mark the paper so you can fold the ends.
4. Unfold the paper and cut along the end creases, taking care not to cut into the middle of the paper.

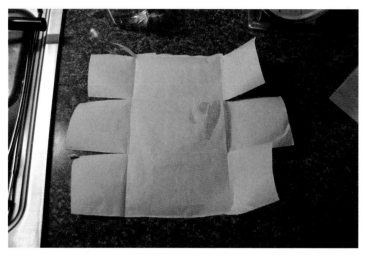

Figure 37.11 Trim as shown.

5. Fold the sides up, similar to wrapping a present.

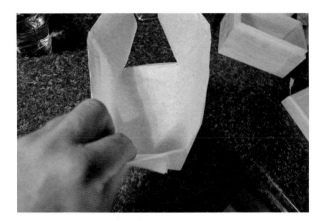

Figure 37.12 Fold each side.

6. Place parchment paper box inside mold.

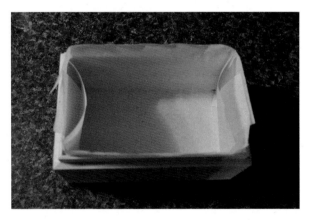

Figure 37.13 Place paper inside box.

7. Alternatively, if you don't mind some crease marks in your final product, you can simply press in some thick plastic wrap and tape it in place.

Note:
   This technique is suitable with other ingredients. Once you have followed this recipe a few times, you can easily find a soap calculator online and try other combinations.

Project 38: DIY Vegetable Rennet

Most cheese was historically made with animal rennet. Nowadays, a lot of cheese is made with mold-based rennet, but it is possible to make a vegetarian rennet for those who are either vegetarian, vegan, or who do not have the resources to make animal-based rennet.

The biggest problem with vegetable rennet is that it becomes bitter in aged cheeses, so it should not be used with raw milk, or cheeses like cheddar that need aging to build their sharp taste.

The plants that can be used with various techniques to make a vegetable-based rennet are:

• Thistle
• Fig
• Yarrow
• Ground ivy
• Lady's Bedstraw
• Nettle
• Pineapple
• Artichoke

Since artichokes and thistles are in the same family, I will show you how to make rennet using them. However, as a rule of thumb, if you crush and extract the sap from the greenery of any of the plants above, you can use it to thicken milk.

Material:

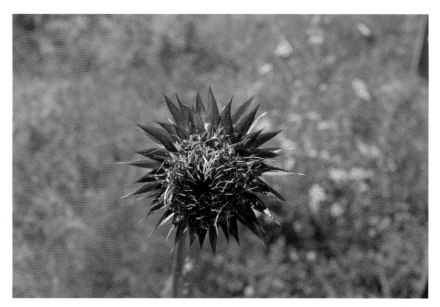

Figure 38.1 Thistle flower

- Thistle flower head when it has turned brown, but harvest it before the plant produces the thistle down, in which case it is too late. Or
- The purple head of the artichoke before it makes the head

Equipment:

- Dehydrator
- Pot

Procedure:

1. Dry the flower heads and pick off the purple stamens.

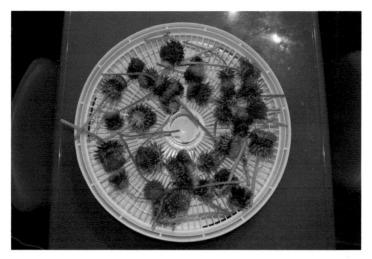

Figure 38.2 Dry the flowers (will take some time).

2. Boil water and drop thistles into the water. Let steep into a thick dark tea.

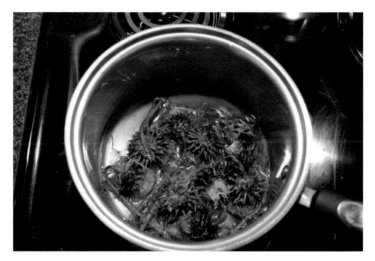

Figure 38.3 Make a dark tea with the thistle heads.

3. Strain off the liquid. This is now thistle flower rennet.

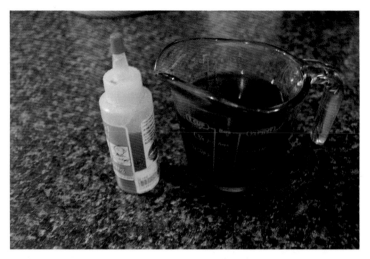

Figure 38.4 The cup contains thistle rennet, the dropper contains commercially made rennet—note the similar color.

4. The rennet can now be added to warmed milk to curdle it and begin the cheese making process.

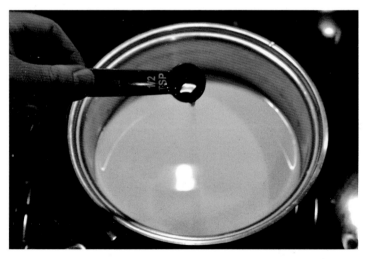

Figure 38.5 Milk curdled with thistle rennet.

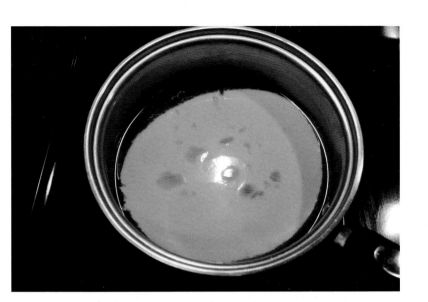

Figure 38.6 The amount of rennet needed will vary
depending on the flowers used.

Note:

Most cheese recipes using commercial rennet are in the teaspoon/
tablespoon amounts. I started using a traditional recipe amount, but
ended up using ½ cup of my homemade rennet to get a good result.

Project 39: Homemade Pectin

Pectin is a natural polysaccharide that, when heated with sugar, creates the thickening effect that is essential to making jams and jellies.

While you can buy pectin at almost any grocery store, it is also quite easily made with tart green apples. Crabapples work best—or Granny Smith if you don't have a crabapple tree—but really any small green and immature apple is likely to work.

This used to be a common skill for homemakers, as making jam and jellies was the best way to preserve fruits for the winter and commercially made pectin was not available.

One thing that the home pectin maker needs to know is that pectin levels vary from plant to plant, and from day to day, so this technique needs to be tested so you can know how much pectin to use in a recipe. We list a method of testing pectin at the end of this project.

There are two things that work in harmony to make jelly jell: the amount of sugar and the strength of the pectin. If you have a low concentration of pectin you will have to use more sugar.

The fruits you are making jelly with also play a role—if you are using fruits with a small amount of natural pectin you will need to boil the mixture until it reduces to almost the same amount of jelly as you started with with natural pectin.

There is definitely a learning curve when using natural pectin, but I find that if you just cannot get something to jell, process it anyway. I use a spoonful of the "jelly" in a glass of water to make a delicious fruit punch. As I write this I am enjoying a glass of blackberry/blueberry/strawberry punch over ice and I may intentionally start canning fruit juice concentrate rather than jelly.

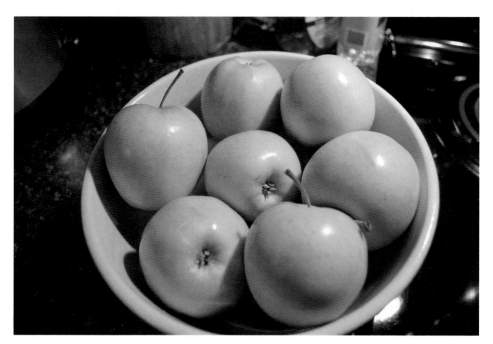

Figure 39.1 The ingredients

Ingredients:

- 3 pounds sliced and washed green apples
- 4 cups water
- 2 tablespoons of lemon juice

Equipment:

- Knife
- Pot
- Measuring cup
- Cheesecloth or jelly bag
- Clean/sanitized mason jar, lid, and ring

Procedure:

1. Wash, but don't peel, the green apples.
2. Cut them into pieces and place in a pot.

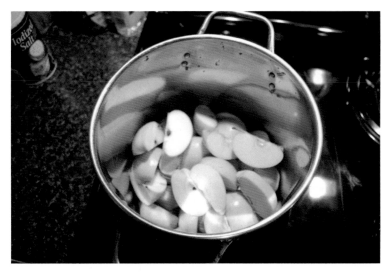

Figure 39.2 Cut and place in a pot with just enough water to cover.

3. Add four cups of water and two tablespoons of lemon juice.

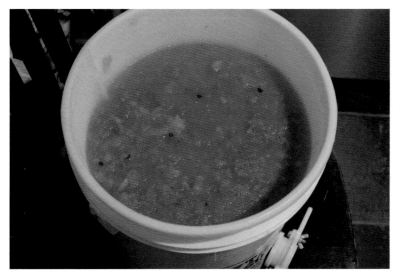

Figure 39.3 Cook all day until mush and strain.

4. Cook on low medium/low until it reduces to a slimy mush. Don't get impatient—this takes a long time.
5. Strain it through cheesecloth or a jelly bag. You can press it to make it drain faster, but that will result in a cloudy and/or apple-flavored end product.
6. Pour it into sanitized jars and can or freeze if desired. It is easy to get a year's supply of pectin in one shot this way.

Yield:
This is an inexact recipe, because the pectin content of the fruit will vary. A general guide is that the riper the fruit, the lower the pectin level. To determine proper use, you will need to perform a jell test.

Bonus Project: Jell Test

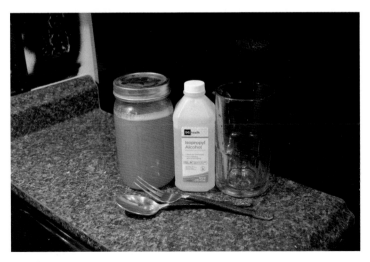

Figure 39.4 Use as strong an isopropyl alcohol as you can get.

When you are making jelly and get to the point where you are about ready to fill the jars, remove a spoonful of the jam and hold an ice cube against the bottom of the spoon to cool the jam.

If the spoonful sets to your liking, then your jelly is ready to be put in jars and processed in the canner.

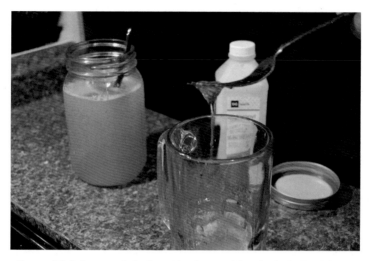

Figure 39.5 A spoonful of pectin dropped in alcohol should gel.

If the spoonful does not set, add another cup of sugar, ¼ cup of lemon juice and more of your pectin. Bring to a full boil for 1 minute and test again.

Store your pectin in a sealed jar in the refrigerator, freezer, or water bath can as you would jelly.

Project 40: Corncob Jelly

This week's project is one that I have seen on many Internet sites and multiple canning and old-school food preservation books. It took me a while to get around to trying it, and when I did I found that the jelly tasted a lot like honey. Honestly, I wish I had done this much sooner.

I typically only cook corn on the cob when grilling out with my family, and when I do so, I tend to cook a lot of corn. This recipe lets me turn the normally wasted water from boiling corn into a tasty food product in itself. Traditionally, red field corn was used to make this recipe, but personally, I have only used sweet corn.

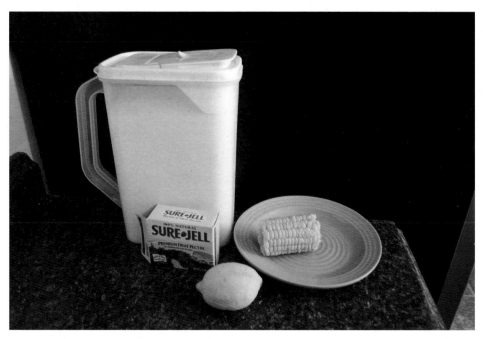

Figure 40.1 The ingredients

Ingredients:

- 12 large ears of corn
- 2 quarts water
- 2 tablespoons lemon juice
- 1 package powdered pectin
- Sugar (amount will vary, but 4–5 cups should be enough)

Equipment:

- Knife
- Measuring cup
- Nonreactive (Steel pot)
- Spoon
- Canning funnel
- Canning jars, lids, rings
- Water bath canner
- Canning jar lifter
- Towel

Procedure:

1. Cook corn, cut kernels from cobs, and store for future use.
2. Measure 2 quarts water into a large pot and add corn cobs.

3. Bring water to a boil and keep uncovered at a rolling boil for 30 minutes to concentrate the liquid.

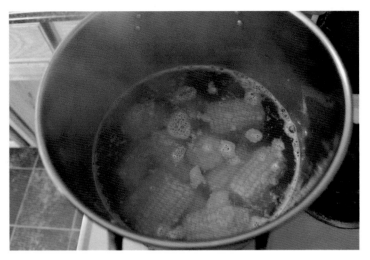

Figure 40.2 Boil corn.

4. I try to boil it down until I get 3 ½–4 cups of liquid.
5. Stir in 2 tablespoons of lemon juice.

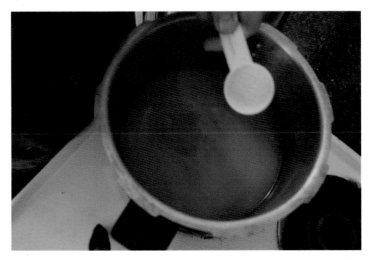

Figure 40.3 Add lemon juice.

6. Add pectin and bring to a boil.

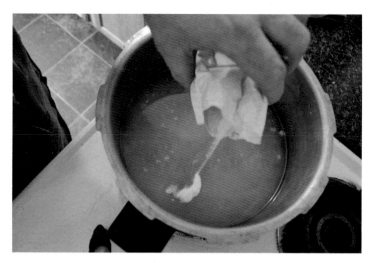

Figure 40.4 Add pectin.

7. Add one cup of sugar per cup of liquid. Stir to dissolve sugar.

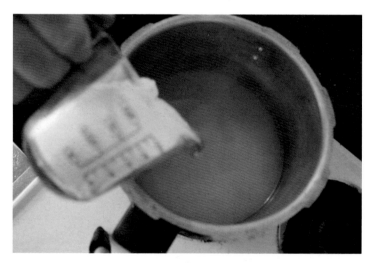

Figure 40.5 Add sugar according to directions on pectin box.

8. Bring pot to a rolling boil. Boil for one minute while stirring constantly.

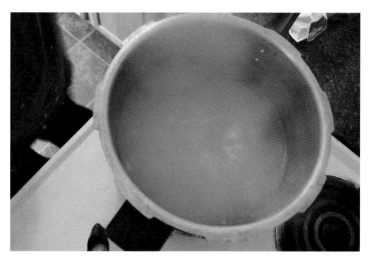

Figure 40.6 Boil for one minute.

9. Remove from heat.
10. Ladle hot corn cob jelly into hot jars.

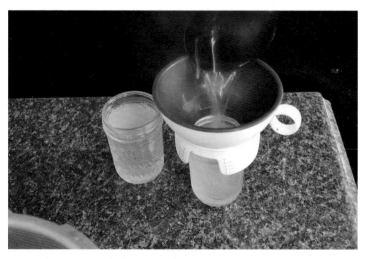

Figure 40.7 Ladle into jars.

11. Adjust lids and bands.

12. Process in a boiling water bath for 10 minutes.

    a.   Add enough water in the canner to cover lids with one inch of water.

    b.   Start time when water is boiling.

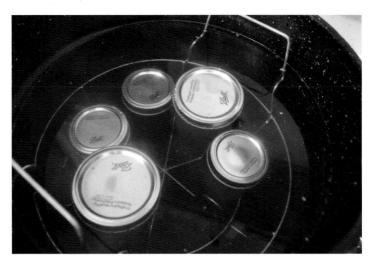

Figure 40.8 Process in a water bath canner.

Yield:

  5 half-pints

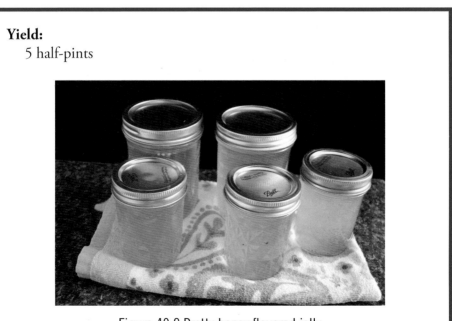

Figure 40.9 Pretty honey flavored jelly

Project 41: Rocket Stove

Being able to sustainably cook and heat is something that every prepper needs to plan for. It is not uncommon for modern homes to rely solely upon electricity for both. Today's project shows you how to use twigs to create a very clean burning stove that provides much heat without having to burn large amounts of wood.

A rocket stove is able to burn efficiently by using high temperature and a good air draft coming from the bottom of the stove. Once the basic premise is understood, these stoves can be quickly built from improvised materials at hand. In this project we will use a #10 can as the base, but I have seen commercially built stoves using 55-gallon drums, or even homebuilt stoves out of stovepipe and rock used to pressure can food at a hunting camp.

Rocket stoves are very fuel efficient, and it is a very scalable technology. After building a small stove like the one in this project, you could easily scale this up to a 55-gallon drum and heat a building.

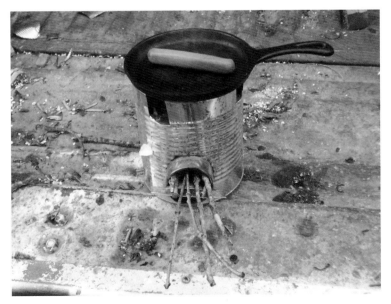

Figure 41.1 Finished rocket stove

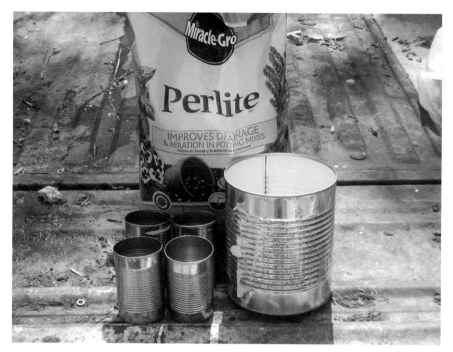

Figure 41.2 The materials

Materials:

- Empty #10 can
- 4 10.5-oz soup/vegetable cans
- Insulation (perlite, sand, dirt, ash—basically any flame resistant insulating material)

Equipment:

- Tin snips
- Hammer
- Pliers
- File
- Gloves
- Drill, punch or nail
- Marker

Procedure:

1. Remove all labels from all the cans and clean cans well.
2. Use one of your cans to trace a circle onto the side of the #10 can. It should be about ½ inch from the bottom of the #10 can.
3. Next, drill, punch, or nail some access holes inside the drawn circle so that you can cut out the circle using your tin snips.
4. Mark and cut a hole in the side of a soup can (can A).

   a. This hole needs to be at the same height as the hole in the #10 can.
   b. It may be best to set the soup can in the #10 can, press it against the hole cut in the larger can and mark the smaller circle through the hole.

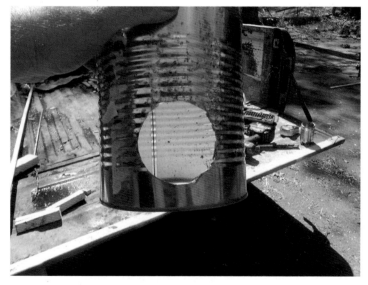

Figure 41.3 Cut a can-sized hole ½ inch from bottom of #10 can.

5. Since this can needs to form an "elbow" with the second soup can (can B), make sure that can B can fit securely in the hole.

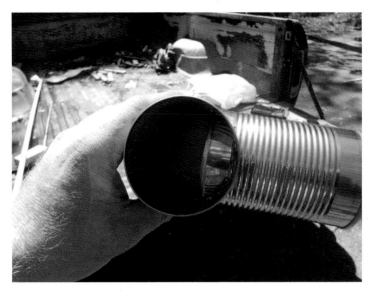

Figure 41.4 Elbow formed by two soup cans

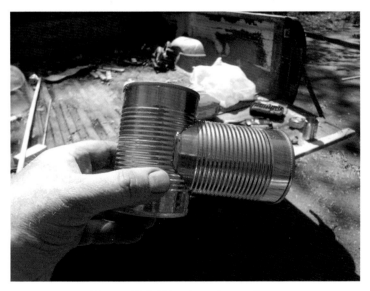

Figure 41.5 Side view of can elbow

6. Cut bottom off soup can (can B) and fit as elbow.

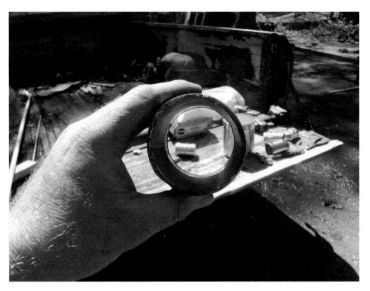

Figure 41.6 Bottom is cut out of soup can B.

7. With can B stuck in can A, use a marker to reach down and mark can B where it meets can A.

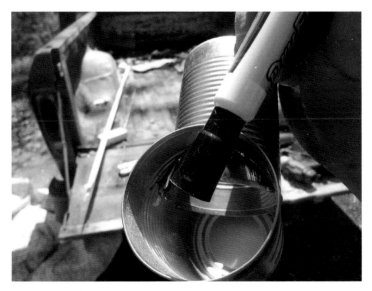

Figure 41.7 Mark where can B meets can A.

8. Cut can B along the mark.

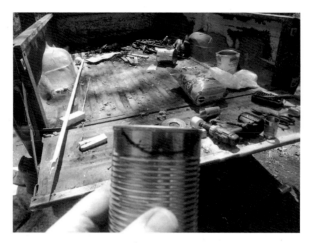

Figure 41.8 Cut along mark.

9. Cut base out of third soup can (can C), and slit the can down the center.
10. Overlap the cut ends of can C so that you can slide it into the soup can elbow. Compare the elbow with the can C chimney, and compare it with the #10 can. Note how much farther the chimney sits above the top of the #10 can.
11. Mark and cut out a half circle of can C (much like how you cut can B). This allows can C to sit deeper in the elbow. The top of the assembly must sit approximately ¼ inch below the edge of the #10 can.

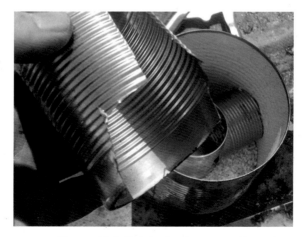

Figure 41.9 Finished cuts on can C

12. Get the lid from the #10 can and cut a hole in the lid so can C can tightly fit through.

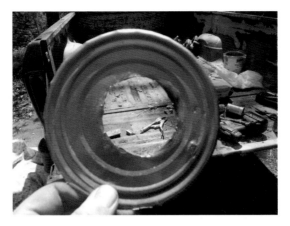

Figure 41.10 Hole cut in #10 can lid

13. Take a can and center it on the #10 can lid, trace the circle, and cut it out with tin snips.
14. Cut eight ½-inch-long slits vertically from the top of the #10 can.
15. To assemble, set can A into the #10 can, ensuring that the open end of can A is facing up.
16. Push can B through the hole cut into the #10 can, and into the hole cut into can A.
17. Can A should be centered into #10 can, with a portion of can B sticking out of the side of the #10 can.

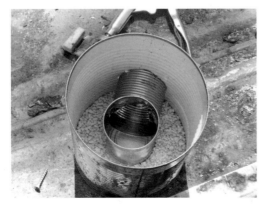

Figure 41.11 Cans A and B inserted in #10 can

18. Push can C into the top of can B, forming a chimney.
19. Fill with insulation material.

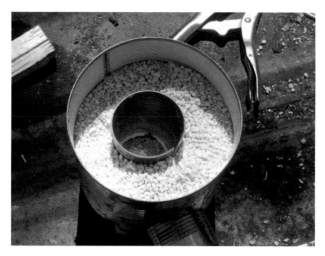

Figure 41.12 Fill with insulation.

20. Insert #10 can lid over chimney formed by can C.
21. Press the lid down slightly.
22. Secure the lid by bending every other tab formed by the ½ slits in the top of the #10 can. This should leave 4 tabs standing up to hold a cooking pot upright.

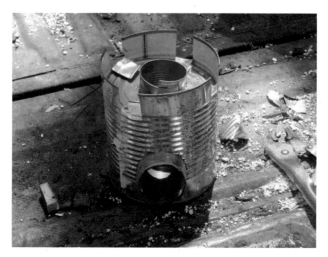

Figure 41.13 Bend tabs down to secure lid in place.

23. The top of the chimney should be below the edge of the 4 upright tabs.
24. Make a fuel shelf from a fourth soup can (can D), cut the can open lengthways, and flatten it out.
25. Cut a "T" shape into the can, with the long leg approximately the size of the width of the center of can B.

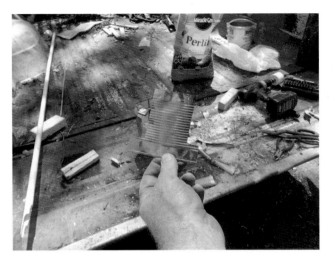

Figure 41.14 Can D should form a "T."

26. Leave "wings" slightly larger to keep the shelf from being pushed into the stove.

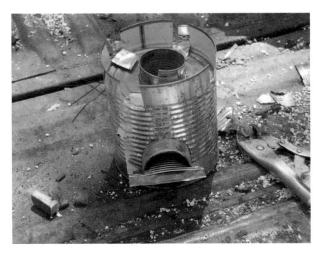

Figure 41.15 Wings keep the "T" in place.

To Light:

1. Wad some paper or tinder, light it, and drop down the chimney.
2. Push small twigs or other kindling-sized fuel into the stove through can B. It should sit on top of the shelf you just cut.
3. Air will flow into the stove through the channel under the shelf.
4. As the fuel burns, push it deeper into the stove so that it can fully combust.

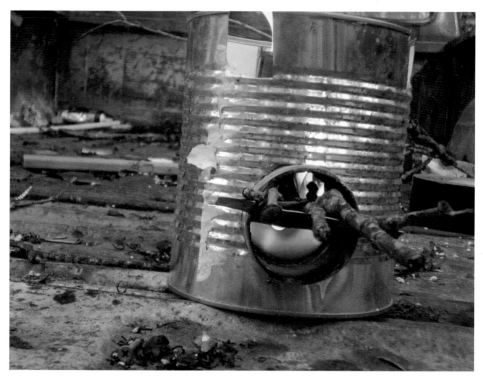

Figure 41.16 Works well, but it gets *hot*.

Project 42: Substituting Honey for Sugar

If you want to eat healthier, or use honey that you have produced yourself, the first thing you need to know is that the rules for sugar substitutions are more like guidelines.

In general, substituting honey for sugar is a matter of preference.

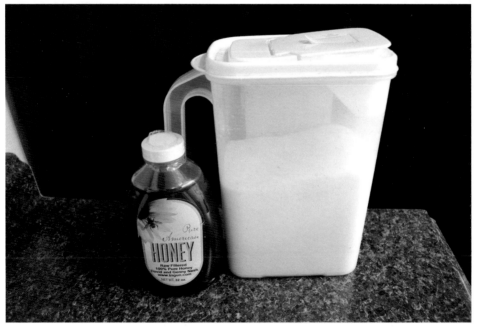

Figure 42.1 Honey for sugar

Some use it cup for cup, others prefer ½ – ⅔ cup of honey per cup of white sugar.

However, because of the water content, reduce the amount of other liquids by ¼ cup for every cup of honey used.

Honey also causes foods to brown much easier, so lower the oven temperature about 25°F to prevent over-browning.

Also, since honey is naturally acidic, and baking soda is a base, add ¼ teaspoon of baking soda for each cup of honey to your recipe.

If you are using the sugar to can, use ⅞ cup of honey for every cup of sugar, but don't change the other liquids. Honey may be substituted effectively for up to half the sugar called for in a canning syrup recipe (test this for jellies).

Remember that honey has its own unique flavor. In general it is a light and pleasing flavor, but if it conflicts with the desired taste of your recipe, there's not much you can do about it. However, the flavor depends on the flowers the bees used to make it, and some flowers give an off taste.

If you are diabetic like I am, keep in mind that honey does not reduce the calorie or carbohydrate content of the sugar syrup, and thus is not an acceptable sugar replacement for people on diabetic diets. However, it is less processed, and there is some evidence that it is a much healthier sweetener in other ways.

You can also use honey as a substitute for other sweeteners:

• Brown Sugar: Follow the same ratio as with substituting honey for table sugar, but replace a portion of the honey with molasses to retain the expected flavor (brown sugar is just unrefined white sugar with the molasses taken out).
• Corn Syrup: Use exactly the same amount, but reduce any other sweet ingredients, since honey has greater sweetening power than corn syrup.
• Molasses: Use exactly the same amount. The resulting flavor and color will be lighter and less heavy. The reverse is true if you swap molasses for honey.

Project 43:
Honey & Vinegar Candy

I added this recipe for several reasons. First, my son loves candy, and I like having "healthy" sweets to give him. Second, it is a good use of honey and vinegar—two things you can easily make yourself (or harvest, in the case of honey). Lastly, if you are ever in a catastrophic disaster where you can neither get, nor afford sweets, you would be surprised by how much a lift a bit of candy can give a person.

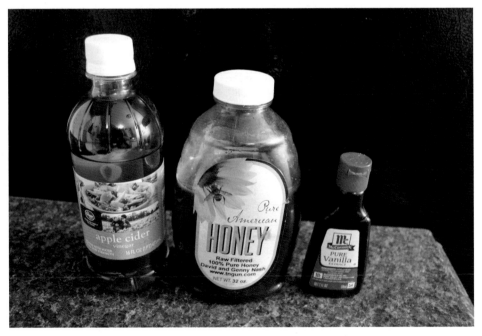

Figure 43.1 The ingredients

Ingredients:

- 1 cup honey
- ¼ cup apple cider vinegar (or fruit-infused vinegar)
- (optional) ½ teaspoon pure vanilla extract

Equipment:

- Heavy saucepan
- Candy thermometer
- Spoon
- Parchment paper
- Baking sheet

Procedure:

1. Pour the honey and vinegar into a heavy saucepan.
2. Place pan over medium heat until mixture starts to boil.
3. Adjust the heat lower if needed and let boil until honey reaches 300°F (hard crack stage).

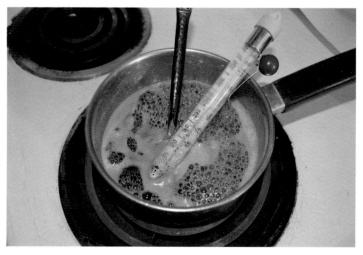

Figure 43.2 Boil gently until mix reaches 300°F.

4. Remove from heat.
5. Add vanilla, if desired.
6. Immediately pour onto a parchment-lined baking sheet.

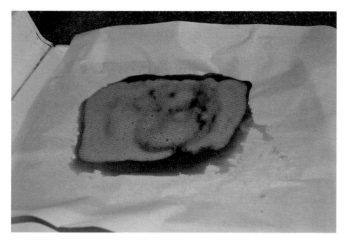

Figure 43.3 Pour 300-degree mix onto parchment-lined cookie sheet.

7. Place in freezer or refrigerator to cool.
8. Once the candy is cooled completely, break into long strips, then break again into small bite-sized pieces.

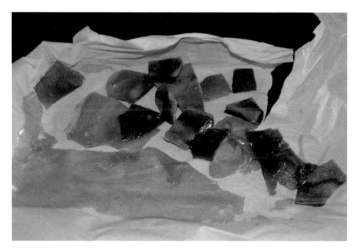

Figure 43.4 Break into bite-sized pieces.

9. Store in freezer.

Yield:
Small ziplock bag of candy

Notes:
Periodically calibrate your candy thermometer by dipping the tip of it in a small pot of boiling water (you can do this while cooking pasta too, as a time saver) and let sit for a few minutes without touching the sides or bottom. It should read 212°F (at sea level). Note any difference in reading and adjust when using. When candy making, following the temperatures listed in the recipe is vital to the quality of the finished product.

Honey can scorch and burn if heated too high.

You can also pour this in sucker molds to make lollipops, but this candy will get chewy rapidly, so it is not a good choice for a small kid's sucker.

If you let the mix cool in your pot, it will become a nightmare to clean, so fill your still-hot pot with warm, soapy water soon after pouring out the candy and let it soak for a while in your sink.

Project 44:
Pepper-infused Honey

The flavor combination of sweet and hot is a favorite of mine. I love chili in my chocolate. When I first heard of honey infused with pepper, I had to try it.

Not only is it simple, but it tastes really good. This is a great recipe to use as a marinade or a glaze.

This is also a way to keep your pepper flavor over the winter, as honey does not spoil.

I look at this as a cousin to candying fruit, which is a traditional food preservation technique that we may experiment with later.

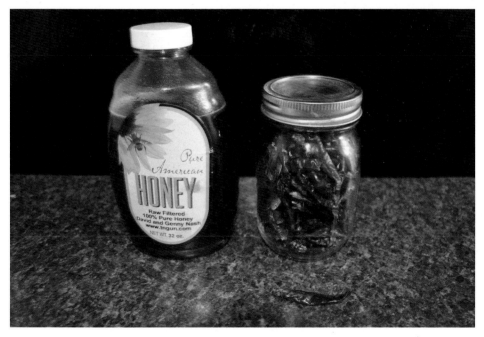

Figure 44.1 The ingredients

Ingredients:

- 1 cup honey
- 3 tablespoons crushed red peppers (about 10 small dried peppers)

Equipment:

- Double boiler (or a glass bowl in a saucepan of boiling water)
- Strainer
- Glass jars

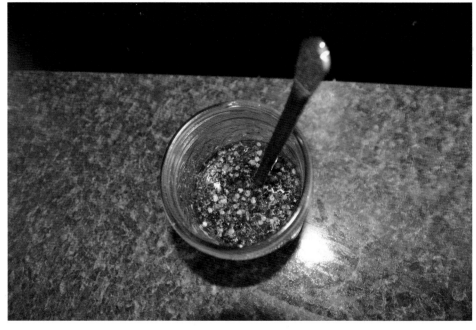

Figure 44.2 Honey/Pepper mix

Procedure:

1. Put the honey into a double boiler.

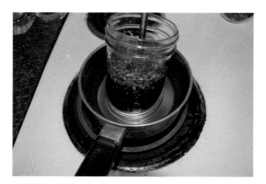

Figure 44.3 Improvised double boiler

2. Heat for 5–10 minutes at about 150°F. A thermometer isn't strictly necessary, but you don't want to destroy the beneficial enzymes in the honey by heating it too high (over 185°F).
3. Turn off the heat and let it steep for about 10 minutes in the double boiler.
4. Strain into a clean jar while the honey is still warm.

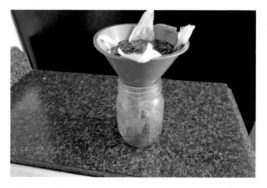

Figure 44.4 Strain the pepper out if desired.

Yield:
One cup of flavored honey

Bonus Project: Roasted Chicken with Pepper Honey Glaze

There is a lot you can do with pepper-infused honey, but using it as a glaze is probably the easiest. At the heart of this recipe, you simply pour honey over a chicken and bake it. The flavor will infuse and the honey will thicken and help hold in some moisture.

When I make honey specifically to make a glaze, I tend not to totally filter out the pepper flakes as I think it enhances the look of the glaze, but that is really up to your personal preference.

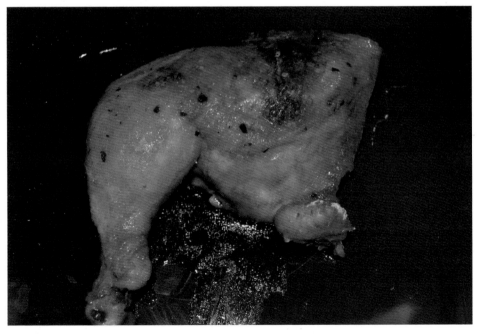

Figure 44.5 Glazed Chicken

Materials:

- 6 chicken thighs
- 2 cups of flour
- 1 pint of pepper-infused honey

Equipment:

- Bowl or ziplock bag
- Baking dish

Procedure:

1. Preheat oven to 350°F.
2. Place flour in bowl or ziplock bag and dredge chicken until lightly coated with flour.
3. Spread chicken out into a single layer in a large baking dish.
4. Cover chicken with half of the infused honey.
5. Bake for 30 minutes.
6. Remove chicken and coat with the rest of the honey.
7. Bake for an additional 10–15 minutes, or until chicken is no longer pink and juices run clear.
8. Let cool 10 minutes before serving.

Yield:
  6 servings of one chicken thigh

Project 45:
Beeswax Food Wrap

Since I work nights, and cannot leave to get food (nor do I want to spend the money), I normally take leftovers to work to eat. This means I use a lot of plastic wrap and aluminum foil to make my food easier to transport.

Using items like plastic wrap and foil is not very frugal, and many people are starting to worry about BPA or other contaminants getting into food from these plastics.

I admit that I'm not all that concerned with this. I figure the mayonnaise will kill me long before plastics will, but I don't like paying for disposable wraps and I like to experiment with new ideas.

When looking up alternatives to plastic wrap, I found several websites selling beeswax-impregnated cotton wraps that take the place of plastic (actually this was the norm *before* plastic wrap) . . .

There are a couple ways to make these wraps, for example, sandwiching the cotton between parchment paper and heating it with an iron, which looks cool. But since my wife has a standing order for me not to use her iron for "experiments" ever again, I will show you the oven method.

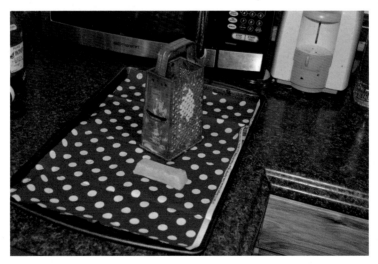

Figure 45.1 The ingredients

Equipment:

- 100 percent cotton cloth (about the thickness of sheets)—I imagine muslin would work but I used a cut-up quilting square.
- Beeswax—I used some from my own beehive, but you can easily find either beeswax ingots or the easier to use beeswax beads in craft stores in the candle making supplies.
- Cookie sheet—once you get hot wax on the sheet, it will forever be useless for baking cookies on. Once again I have project cooking utensils and food cooking utensils because I do *not* like being hit about the head and neck with a rolling pin . . .
- Grater (if using solid beeswax ingots)

Procedure:

1. Preheat your oven to 170–190°F. Beeswax is highly flammable and melts between 143 and 151°F so don't try to overheat it to speed up the process (unless you want to call the insurance adjuster).
2. Cut your cloth to the desired size (this is up to you). You can hem the edges or use pinking shears to make a nice edge, but I just whacked at it with an old pair of scissors.
3. If using ingots, grate them using your cheese grater. If using beads you can skip this step.
4. Set your cloth in the cookie sheet and lightly dust with the bits of wax— you want an even coat.

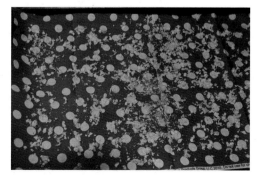

Figure 45.2 Cover lightly and evenly with wax chips.

5. Less wax will let more moisture pass though, while more wax makes a stiffer cloth.
6. Put the cookie sheet with the cotton and wax into the oven. Five minutes will do just fine. A longer time may cause problems, so if it is not all melted at 5 minutes keep a very watchful eye. You don't want to scorch your cloth or ignite the wax.
7. After you take the cloth out of the oven, immediately remove from the cookie sheet and hang to cool. It should appear darker. Any light spots did not receive as much wax, so be on the lookout for this.

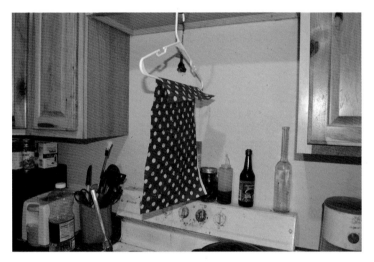

Figure 45.3 After the wax melts, hang it to dry.

8. Once cool you can use immediately. You can wrap sandwiches with this directly, or, if you use more wax to make a stiffer cloth, you can actually wrap this over a plate to cover it.

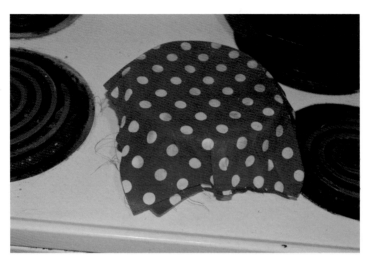

Figure 45.4 The stiff cloth can cover plates directly.

If your wrap gets dirty, you can easily clean it with cold water. Don't use soap or hot water as this will impact your wax.

Project 46:
How to Make a Zeer Pot

Your mileage may vary with this project; it is touted in appropriate technology circles as a wonderful alternative to a refrigerator. I find that it does not work as well as it could here in the humid South. I would imagine that since the cooling works through evaporation, it would do much better in the southwestern United States than it does in my home state of Tennessee.

However, it is bone simple to do, and relatively cheap, and since it works enough to keep a few water bottles comfortably cool sitting next to the lawn chair I figure even if it's not perfect in every location, the technology is worth sharing.

Zeer Pot technology is used in some very poor countries to reduce food spoilage. It is also the technology behind Latin American ceramic water crocks called Olas which provide cool drinking water in hot arid conditions.

All a zeer pot is, is a simple fridge made of local materials. It is one earthenware pot set inside another, with a layer of wet sand in between. As the moisture evaporates it cools the inner pot, keeping up to 12 kg of fruit and vegetables fresher for longer.

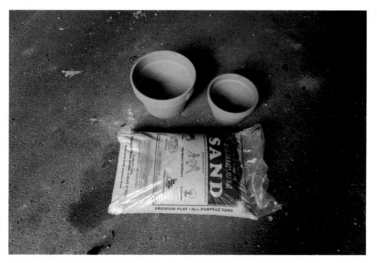

Figure 46.1 The materials

Materials:

- Two unglazed ceramic pots—terra cotta pots seem to work best. The smaller inner pot holds your food items, so size appropriately. The outer pot needs to be larger. (I use a pot two sizes bigger than the inner pot so I have room to pack in a lot of sand.)
- Fine white sand (play sand from the hardware store works well)
- Tape, plastic disks or some other method to plug the hole in the outer pot so the sand does not leak out (or set it on a coaster and do not move it)
- Towel
- Water

Procedure:

1. Stop up the hole in the large pot with some tape (coffee filters work best)

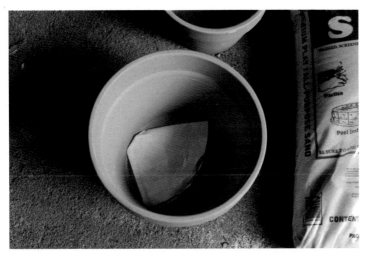

Figure 46.2 Stop up the hole in the bottom of the pot.

2. Fill the bottom of the large pot with just enough sand so that the small pot can sit inside and the tops of both pots are flush with each other.

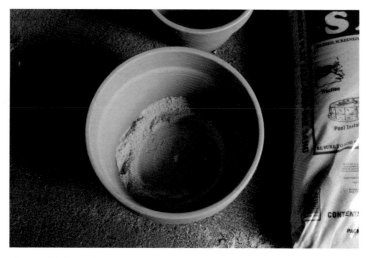

Figure 46.3 Fill bottom with enough sand so that the smaller pot will fit flush with the top of the outer pot.

3. Center the small pot inside the larger one.
4. Fill the space between the two ceramic pots with a loose layer of sand.

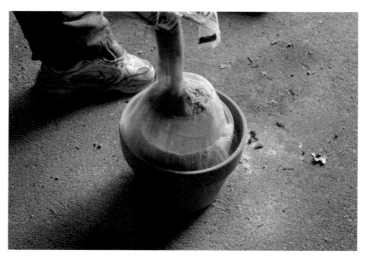

Figure 46.4 It's easiest to fill if you upend a bowl over the small pot and pour the sand over it.

5. Gently pour some water in the sand to thoroughly moisten it and the inner pot.
6. Insert whatever you want to keep cool in the inner pot.

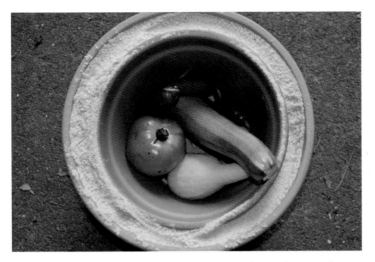

Figure 46.5 Fill with fruit and cover with a moist towel.

7. Cover the whole assembly with a wet towel.

Notes:

This process works by evaporation, so you will need to keep the sand and the towel damp (not sopping wet). This also means it works best on dry hot days.

It does not cool your food like a refrigerator would, but it does have a nice temperature difference. I have seen many people get temperature differences of up to 20°F in ideal conditions.

During the Crusades, Saladin was able to use this technology (along with specially designed shade buildings) to get ice in the desert, which greatly impressed King Richard.

Project 47: Freezing Fruits and Vegetables

In my opinion, surviving is easiest when you have appropriate skills and are open to using the best possible techniques—that means you are comfortable using proven techniques from history as well as adopting appropriate new technology.

Freezing food is relatively new, but it revolutionized how households are fed.

Unfortunately, there is more to freezing food for long term than just tossing food in the freezer and thawing them out at a later time.

When water freezes, it crystallizes. So when the water in food freezes it breaks the cell walls of the food. Since the cells walls provide structure to the plants, fruits and vegetables get mushy when they thaw.

There are several ways to reduce this damage, and in this week's project I will show you many of them.

One of the ways to reduce the amount of damage is to freeze foods as quickly as possible, as colder temperatures produce smaller crystals, which in turn cause less damage to cells. Alternatively, you can just eat fruit before it completely thaws. Half thawed fruit will mask the "mushy" texture.

Some foods freeze better than others; for example, low acid vegetables freeze much better than high acid foods like tomatoes. Luckily, high acid foods can better than low acid vegetables, so flexibility is key.

Blanching vegetables, by very quickly submerging them in boiling water, and then quenching them in ice cold water will prevent naturally occurring enzymes in the food from damaging color, flavor, and nutrients. Inspecting fruit and vegetables before freezing to discard damaged food also helps maintain good quality.

If you are freezing cut fruits that brown (like apples, bananas, peaches, or apricots), treat with vitamin C—a quick dip in a bowl of water with a little lemon juice added will prevent browning. I use a mix of one quart water to a tablespoon of lemon juice.

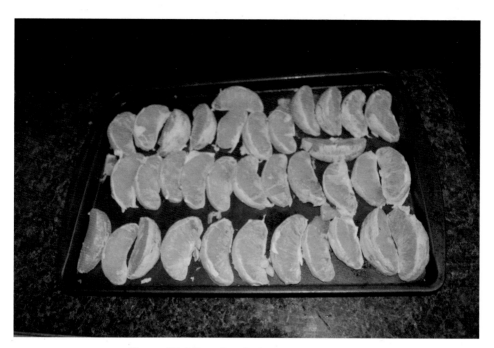

Figure 47.1 Freezing fruits as a single layer

When packing, you need to prevent as much air contact as possible to prevent freezer burn. Packing vegetables tightly helps avoid contact; however, if you freeze food that is packed tightly, you will have to thaw the entire batch to use it. I have found that freezing fruits like strawberries or blackberries in a single layer on a baking sheet allows them to freeze individually, so that when packed in a ziplock bag, I can remove just the right amount for my recipe without impacting the rest.

When it is time to use your frozen food, you should know that most food can cook in boiling water when taken straight out of the freezer, but some items like corn need to thaw a bit first. Fruits should be thawed slowly; however, fragile fruits like strawberries will thaw into a mushy consistency, so they are best used as toppings or ingredients in other recipes.

You can store frozen vegetables for a couple years if you prevent freezer burn by tightly packing in an air- and moisture-tight container, but food quality is best if used in under a year. If you're like me, you probably have at least one freezer bag in your freezer of five-year-old squash or beans . . .

Project 48: Storing Eggs Without Refrigeration

By now you may think I am a little obsessed with finding multiple ways to do things, and that may be true, but I find that having skill redundancies works to my advantage more often than not. Earlier, I demonstrated how to pickle eggs to preserve them, and now we are going to try a method to preserve uncooked eggs for months without a fridge to stick them in.

This is a great way to extend the shelf life of eggs, but it does have some drawbacks. First, this method interferes with the ability for an egg to be whipped, so you can't use it for cakes and the like. Second, there is also a process to select the eggs, and a time frame for completing the process that you need to follow.

You need to understand that eggs are pretty robust. You can store them for up to two to three months without doing anything to them if the temperature is lower than 55°F and the humidity is near 75 percent. If humidity levels are too low, the eggs will dry out. If they are too high, the eggs will get moldy.

If you need to store them longer than that, select clean, uncracked eggs that have not been out of the chicken longer than 24 hours (so no store-bought eggs need apply). If an egg is dirty and you need to clean it, then do so, but use that egg for something else since washing it removes the natural protective coating on the egg. If you wash this off, bacteria can more easily enter the egg.

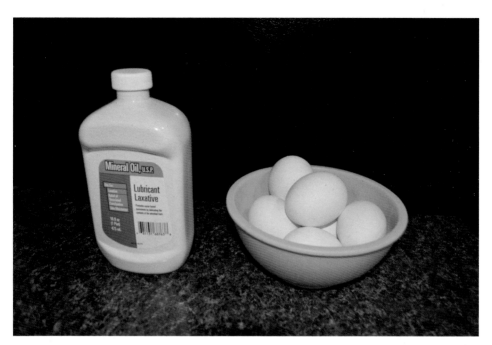

Figure 48.1 The ingredients

Ingredients:

- Eggs
- Mineral oil

Equipment:

- Pot
- Slotted spoon or tongs

Procedure:

1. Pasteurize your mineral oil to ensure that it is free of mold spores or bacteria. To do this, heat it to 180°F for about 20 minutes.

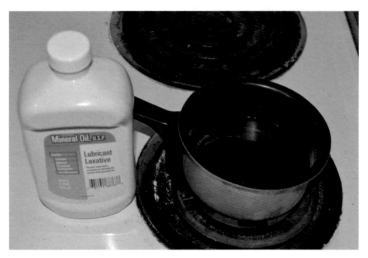

Figure 48.2 Pasteurize your oil.

2. With tongs or a slotted spoon, dip room temperature eggs one at a time into the oil.

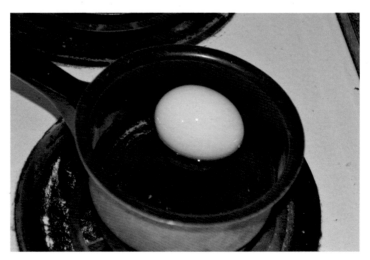

Figure 48.3 Dip room temperature eggs in oil.

3. Set them aside on a rack, such as is used in candy making, and let them drain for about 30 minutes.
4. Pack them away in clean, dry cartons.

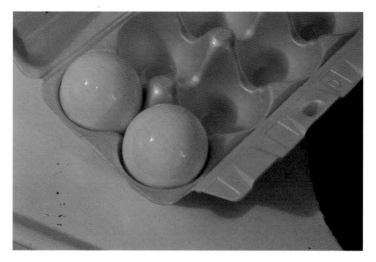

Figure 48.4 Pack in clean cartons.

Place the oiled eggs in a clean, closed carton that is stored in a cool dry place. Coating the egg with oil seals the shell to prevent evaporation during storage. Eggs dipped in oil will keep for several months. However, if stored for too long they will acquire an off flavor, which becomes more pronounced after four months.

Project 49: Pickling Eggs

I am a firm believer in the chicken as an essential homestead animal. They are great scavengers, produce eggs and meat, and, unlike other small animals that are raised for meat, there are few cultural bias against eating them. They are also more common today as their presence in suburbia is becoming more and more acceptable.

Young chickens lay approximately one egg a day. You also need to keep more than one chicken as they are social animals. These two facts together mean that eggs can very quickly overrun your kitchen if you are not careful.

In looking for things to do with eggs I learned three things: First, there are lots of recipes for pickled eggs, and from this I infer that many people like them. Second, I have learned that pickling eggs is pretty easy to do. Lastly, I found several official US government websites that tell me there are no safe ways to can pickled eggs for long-term storage, because one guy got botulism poisoning in 1997.

I don't worry about the botulism risk because I am not canning these for long-term storage. While I know that the temperatures in my canner won't 100 percent kill any botulism spores in the center of my egg, I know that the naturally raised eggs are pretty resistant to letting contaminants through the shell (some people believe that washing them aggressively can help "push" bacteria through the shell). I am not going to go that far, but the egg is a protective coating for a baby and is designed to keep them safe. For botulism spores to grow in the center of an egg stuck in a sealed can, there has to be botulism already present inside the center of the egg. Frankly, I don't see this as being likely, but since it is possible you need to use your own judgment according to what you feel is safe.

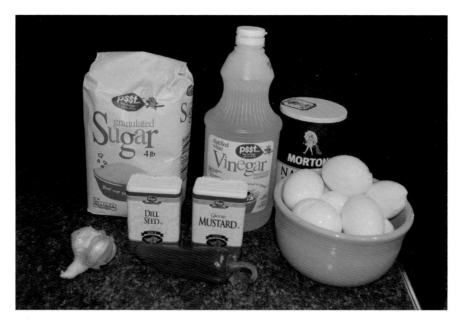

Figure 49.1 The ingredients

Ingredients:

- 2 cups vinegar (5% acidity)
- 2 tablespoons canning Salt
- 1 tablespoon sugar
- ½ teaspoon dill seed
- ¼ teaspoon ground mustard
- 1 clove garlic sliced into thin slices
- 1 jalapeno sliced into thin slices
- 12 peeled hardboiled eggs

Equipment:

- Pot
- Measuring cup and spoons
- Mason jars with sterile lids and rings
- Canning funnel
- Ladle

Procedure:

1. Mix all the ingredients except for eggs in a pot and bring to a boil.

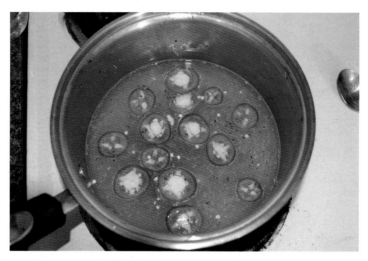

Figure 49.2 Mix all ingredients except eggs and bring to a boil.

2. Once a boil has been reached, let it boil for 3–4 minutes and remove from heat.
3. Strain the jalapeno and garlic from the brine and drop in the bottom of the jars.

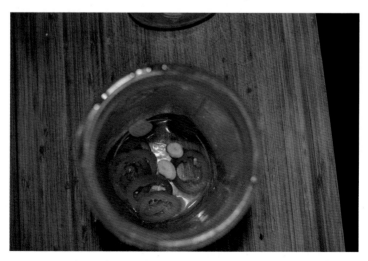

Figure 49.3 Place garlic and pepper slices in bottom of jar.

4. Peel 12 eggs and pack into quart jars on top of the jalapeno and garlic slices.

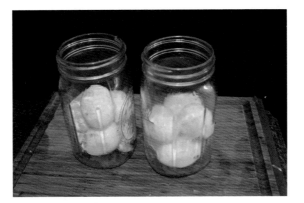

Figure 49.4 Fill jar with peeled eggs.

5. Stir the brine well to make sure the salt is well suspended, then pour the hot brine over the eggs into the jar, leaving ½ inch of head space from the top.
6. Place lid tightly on jar and shake.
7. Refrigerate for 1–10 days and shake the jars slightly each day to keep the pickling mix suspended in solution.

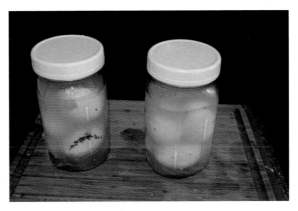

Figure 49.5 Finished eggs

Yield:
   12 pickled eggs

Project 50:
How to Store Potatoes

A lot of folks (like my lovely wife) simply dump a store-bought bag of potatoes in their favorite spot in the kitchen and expect the potatoes to be good until used. Unfortunately that is not always the case.

Potatoes need to be stored in a cool, dark place away from fruits like apples. Apples give off a gas that tells potatoes to rot.

Do not store potatoes in the refrigerator or the starch will convert to sugar, which changes the taste and the consistency (as well as makes your French fries turn dark when cooking).

When potatoes are exposed to the light they also create a toxin. Many know that the light turns potatoes green, and I used to think the green was the toxin and felt I could just peel it away. Turns out, the green color comes at the same time as the poison develops and is merely an indicator—the actual toxins are not in the green parts. Don't eat green potatoes, but feel free to eat green eggs and ham . . .

If you want to grow your own potatoes, follow these steps when harvesting to get the longest storing tubers:

1. Once the plant dies it should be pretty obvious that the potatoes won't get any bigger and are ready for harvest.
2. Don't harvest immediately, but leave them under the ground for a couple more weeks to toughen them up for storage (unless it's going to rain a lot, in which case dig them up before they rot).
3. Look for the base of the plant, then dig several inches away from the base. Look for four to eight potatoes per plant.
4. If you stab a potato with your shovel, separate those and eat them first.

5. Spread a single layer of taters on a newspaper or sheet in a dark room.

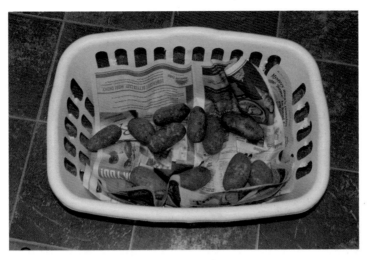

Figure 50.1 Single layer sitting on newspaper

6. Cover them with another newspaper or sheet and let them sit for a week. This causes the skins to toughen up for storage.

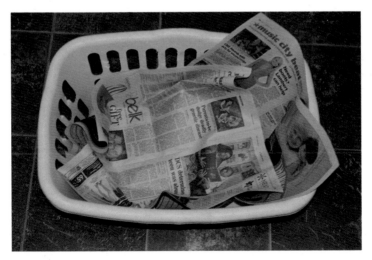

Figure 50.2 Cover with newspaper and repeat until full or out of potatoes.

7. Next, put them in covered boxes or baskets in a dark, cool room.
8. Occasionally sift through your potatoes to check for any that may be rotting. One rotten potato can cause the whole box to rot.
9. If you don't grow your own, you can make your store-bought taters last longer if you line plastic laundry baskets with newspapers, arrange your potatoes in layers between sheets of newspapers, and place the packed, covered baskets in an unheated garage or basement.

Project 51:
Homemade Pasta / Easy Way to Cut Pasta

At first glance, you may wonder how a pasta recipe made it into a prepper/ food preservation book. As an advocate for the storage of bulk wheat, I find it important to give you some recipes for wheat. Let's face it, as great as homemade bread is, bread for every meal can get *boring*! However, I could go a long time eating pasta without experiencing appetite fatigue.

This is a very basic recipe, and a good place to start experimenting with pasta-making techniques. Basically, it is one cup flour to one cup egg with some water to bind.

This recipe is so simple that you don't even need a bowl if you don't mind mixing it directly on your countertop (my lovely bride requires me use a bowl).

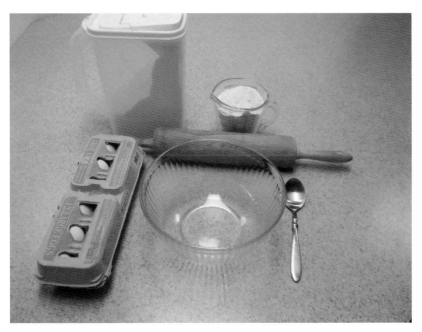

Figure 51.1 The ingredients

Ingredients:

- 1 cup flour (all-purpose works, but high protein, durum-based flours give a hardier finished texture)
- 1 egg
- Water (a small amount may be needed to help shape the dough)

Equipment:

- Rolling pin
- Knife
- Mixing bowl optional

Procedure:

1. Dump flour on counter (or a bowl if you live with a spoil-sport). Make an indention in the center of the pile.
2. Break the eggs into the center of the depression. Gently beat eggs, and slowly move outward, incorporating the flour bit by bit until you end up with a ball of dough. Depending on the weather, the flour, the size of the eggs, and luck; you may need to add a small bit of water to totally form the dough.

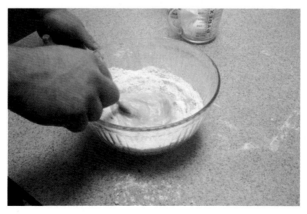

Figure 51.2 Mix well.

3. Once you have a ball of dough, dump it out onto a large floured surface.
4. Knead the dough thoroughly. You want to really work the gluten in the wheat. It will become smooth and take on a consistency a lot like play dough.
5. Using a rolling pin, roll your dough out until it is as thin as you can make it. Pasta will plump as it cooks, so take that into consideration. It is nice if you can keep your dough roughly rectangular in shape, but I always give up as I try to keep it thin.

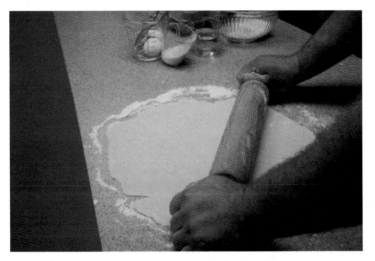

Figure 51.3 Roll your dough thin.

6. You can cut your dough by hand (great if you have patience and attention to detail and want very thin strips). This is most easily done with a pizza cutter or very large dough knife; but I have an easier way.

7. Once you get your dough as thin as you desire, simply roll it into a tube, and, using a sharp knife, slice it as thin as you want.

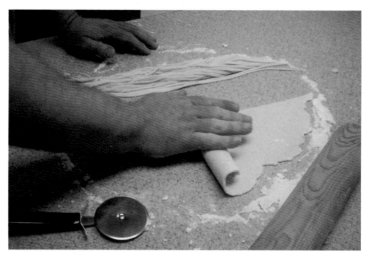

Figure 51.4 Roll it into a tube.

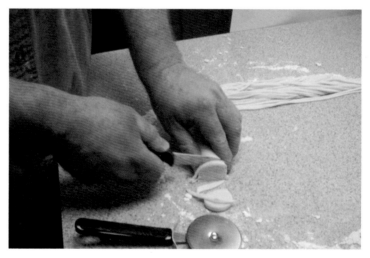

Figure 51.5 Slice as thin as possible.

8. Once you get the dough cut into spirals, simply unroll each spiral into a long noodle, and either dry or cook immediately.

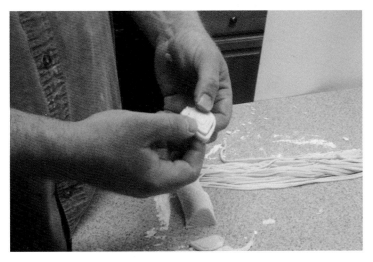

Figure 51.6 Unroll your pinwheel of cut dough.

9. You could dry the noodles for later by hanging them up. They make special drying racks made of small wood dowels, but I think pasta is much tastier if cooked fresh.
10. To cook fresh pasta, simply dump the noodles in the water and they will cook in 2–3 minutes.
11. Drain and serve with whatever sauce you like best.

Yield:

The yield depends on the amount of pasta you make, but a simple 1 cup flour/one egg batch feeds two adults.

Note:

As a rule of thumb, fresh pasta works best for butter sauces and dried pasta is best for sauces with an olive oil base.

Project 52: Hominy (Nixtamalized Corn)

This project looks deceptively simple, but it is one that I had to try a couple times to get right. I only stuck with it because Nixtamalization is a vital process for people who use corn as a staple food. This is because the nutrient niacin is unavailable in unprocessed corn, and by cooking dried corn with a strong alkali (nixtamaling it), niacin becomes available, thereby preventing nutrient deficiency diseases like pellagra.

Besides preventing the typical symptoms of pellagra (diarrhea, dermatitis, dementia and death), this process is how masa (corn tortillas), hominy, grits, and posole are made. This makes the process an essential skill for any culture that is based on corn.

Nixtamalization is simply the process of cooking corn with alkaline, which dissolves the hull and improves the nutritional content of the corn.

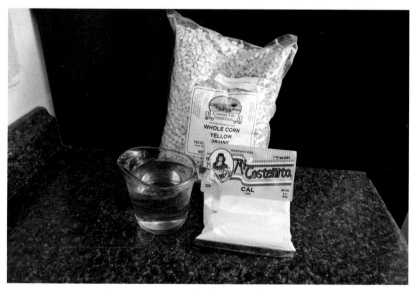

Figure 52.1 The ingredients

Ingredients:

- 2 cups dried corn
- 6 cups water
- 2 tablespoons calcium hydroxide

Equipment:

- Nonreactive pot (stainless steel, borosilicate glass (pyrex), or an unbroken enameled pot)—do *not* use aluminum.
- Nonreactive spoon (I use a wood or plastic spoon)

Procedure:

1. Obtain your calcium hydroxide. You could make lye from wood ashes, but I buy mine at the local Hispanic grocery store. It is sold as "Cal" and is normally on a rack with dried peppers and spices.

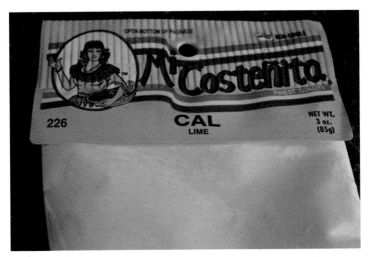

Figure 52.2 Cal

2. Mix the corn, water, and cal and put the pot on medium-low.

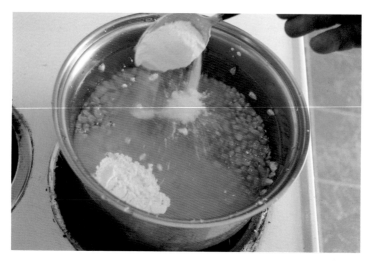

Figure 52.3 Mix and bring to a boil.

3. Slowly bring the mix to a boil (this should take 30–45 minutes). When it boils, remove from heat and let the pot sit overnight.

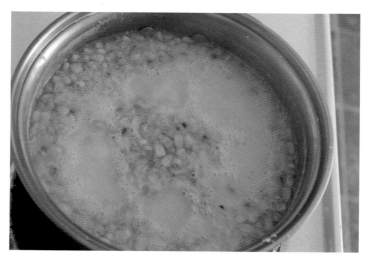

Figure 52.4 Let sit overnight.

4. As the lime chemically alters the corn, the hulls undergo a visible change and loosen.

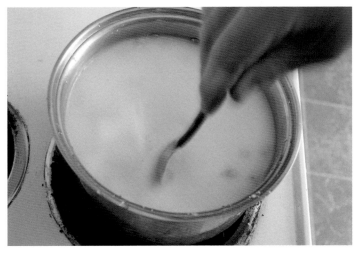

Figure 52.5 The water and corn will change over time as the Cal works.

5. The next day, pour away the cooking liquid and rinse the corn in multiple changes of water.
6. In a bowl full of water, rub the corn in your hands to loosen the hulls.
7. Fill the bowl of corn with water and pour off any pieces of hull that float to the top, then drain.

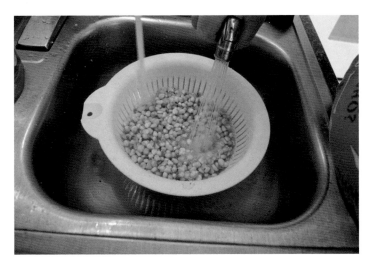

Figure 52.6 The hulls will have a soapy texture and will take a lot of water to rinse away.

8. The dehulled corn is now nixtamilized. It can be ground into masa flour, or dried and broken up into grits.

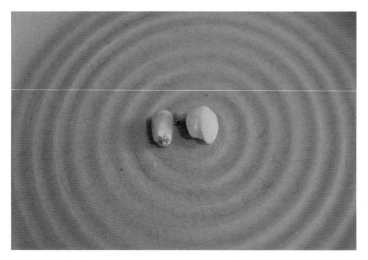

Figure 52.7 Dried corn on left, nixtamilized corn is on right.

Yield:
Approximately 3.5 cups of corn

Notes:
Whan making masa flour the corn is ground wet, using the retained water from the cooking as the liquid component. It is then dried and stored.

When making tortillas from masa flour, add water to the dried masa flour as necessary until the dough begins to form.

Grits are made from dried nixtamilized corn that has been ground into small, rice-sized chunks.

Summary

After completing the projects in this book, you should come away with two things that are worth much more than the price of this book—new skills and an increased level of confidence.

Not everyone has it in them to go out and try to learn new things, much less do so week after week. I truly hope that you would never *have* to use any of the food preservation skills presented in the book in a time of hardship. But I hope you realize the value of being able to, if the convenience of grocery stores on every corner ever became unavailable.

Thank you for reading this book, and I hope you continue on the journey to acquire more skills and knowledge, as we never know when any bit of random knowledge is going to be needed.

About the Author

David is a longtime kitchen experimenter. If you are looking for him and he is not writing or piddling in his workshop, then he is most likely in the kitchen throwing potato peels on the ceiling or dumping flowers on the floor.

While David's loving wife, Genny, appreciates his cooking, that appreciation does not extend to either the messes he creates while cooking, or the occasional kitchen fire.

This is David's third nonfiction work, and his second project book. The first, *52 Prepper Projects*, gained the attention of National Geographic where he was featured on the Season III finale of *Doomsday Preppers*.